HISTORY

OF

AMERICAN MEDICAL LITERATURE

FROM 1776 TO THE PRESENT TIME

BY

S. D. GROSS, M.D

"The chief glory of every people arises from its authors."—DR. JOHNSON.

BURT FRANKLIN
NEW YORK

Published by LENOX HILL Pub. & Dist. Co. (Burt Franklin)
235 East 44th St., New York, N. Y. 10017
Originally Published: 1876
Reprinted: 1972
Printed in the U. S. A.

S.B.N.: 8337-1466X
Library of Congress Card Catalog No.: 72-78009
Burt Franklin: Bibliography and Reference Series 451
American Classics in History and Social Science 238

Reprinted from the original edition in the University
of Pennsylvania Library.

PREFACE.

The matter comprised in the following pages was read as an Introductory Address to the Fifty-first Course of Lectures in the Jefferson Medical College, October 4th, 1875, and published at the request of the Class. It is now issued in a separate form for distribution among my professional brethren, and such persons as may feel a desire to peruse it. The composition cost me much labor, but it was a labor of love, designed to show our people how much earnest work we have done during the century now about to close of our existence as an independent power in the interests of medical science, and in upholding the national honor. Like Rousseau's Ode to Posterity, the booklet may never reach its destination; but if it should be so fortunate, it may, perchance, serve as a connecting link between the glorious Past and what a hundred years hence will undoubtedly be a grand and brilliant Present.

PHILADELPHIA,
Nov. 4th, 1875.

HISTORY OF AMERICAN MEDICAL LITERATURE.

1. INTRODUCTORY REMARKS.

In opening the fifty-first course of lectures in this school, I desire to spend the hour allotted to me for this purpose in the discussion of a subject which, it seems to me, is eminently appropriate to the occasion. Half a century has passed since this school came into existence, and we are on the eve of the anniversary of our national independence. In a few months more the clock of Time will strike the hour of twelve, and usher in the birth of a new century for forty millions of freemen, living in peace and happiness, literally their own governors and their own legislators. We, a portion of this immense hive of human beings, representing almost every nationality on the habitable globe, are assembled here this evening to see what the century, now rapidly passing away, has done for our great profession, and what, in turn, the incoming one has a right to expect from you. Of your speaker, and of others like him, little more is to be expected; they are but links between the past and the present; and any light which they may have emitted will soon be obscured, if not lost, in the dim future. What magic horoscope shall pierce its womb?

The theme which I have selected for my discourse is, "The Progress of American Medical Literature during the last Century;" a theme which, while it may, I think, incite your ambition, will afford us an opportunity of discharging a debt of gratitude to our predecessors and contemporaries; men who have advanced the interests of the profession and surrounded it with a halo of glory. I have undertaken this task, difficult as it is, the more willingly because my entrance into the profession fifty years ago was coeval with the birth of our medical literature. I may add that of some of the authors of whom it will be my province to speak, I was a pupil, that upwards of a score have been my colleagues in medical schools, that many of them have been my personal friends, and that some have been educated under my own teaching.

The first question which naturally presents itself is, Have we a medical literature; and, if so, is it worthy of us as a great profession, and worthy of your acceptance as a guide to the study and practice of the healing art? It is within the recollection of men still living that a writer in the Edinburgh Review, generally supposed to have been Sydney Smith, sneeringly asked, "Who reads an American book?" and, although the remark was not designed to apply especially to professional works, it was not without its significance even here. If the reverend critic, who owed this country a bitter grudge on account of his losses as a Pennsylvania bondholder, could rise from his grave, and stroll through the vast bookstores which would everywhere meet his eye, it is evident that he would change his mind: for it may safely be affirmed that no nation on the globe has made greater or more brilliant progress in general, and even in professional literature, than ours since the utterance of those sarcastic words. It has been well observed by Dr. Johnson, that the chief glory of every people arises from its authors.

When the tocsin of war was sounded on this continent in 1775, by the rebels in arms against the mother country, the physician might have looked around in vain for a native medical book. The whole stock in trade was comprised in a few pamphlets on smallpox, measles, and scarlatina. Our literary and professional works, like our tea and coffee, sugar, and finer fabrics, came from Europe, especially England. Our dependence was absolute. In all the country there was but one medical school; and even this was soon suspended, the lecture-room having been exchanged for the hospital, and the lancet for the sword. There was work to be done. Three millions of human beings, groaning under the yoke of tyranny and oppression, were to be freed: the bond stipulated for blood; the professor's gown was replaced by the epaulette; and for seven long years, alternately marked by hope and despondency, silence reigned supreme in the halls of literature and science. Nor was there any improvement in this respect for a number of years after the struggle had ended. Men could not at once return to their accustomed habits and occupations. The country was impoverished, and heavily in debt. Men had to provide bread for their families. One man alone, of towering intellect and of untiring industry, stood forth during all this period in the midst of his fellow-citizens, like the morning star, gilding the horizon with the effulgence of his genius. Tract after tract fell in rapid succession from his prolific pen, inaugurating thus a new era, and setting in motion a ball destined to roll onward and upward through all the ages on this mighty continent. Benjamin Rush, a farmer's son, born within thirty miles of Philadelphia, a signer of the Declaration of Independence, and at first physician, and then surgeon of the continental army, is the father not only of American Medicine, but of American Medical Literature, the type of a great man, many-sided, far-seeing, full of intellect and genius; abused and vilified, as man hardly ever was before, by his contemporaries, professional and non-professional; misunderstood by his immediate successors, and unappreciated by the present generation, few of whom know anything of his real character. In awarding to this great and good man this high honor, I am but rendering a bare act of justice to his memory. Rush inspired his pupils with ambition, and taught them how to think, for he was facile princeps, "head and shoulder" above all his compeers as a medical philosopher.

These tracts were at length, namely, in 1788–9, collected and published in book form, under the title of "Medical Inquiries and Observations," in four volumes. The treatise upon "Diseases of the Mind," incorporated long ago into the medical literature of Europe, was issued in 1812, and is an enduring monument of his experience, genius, and erudition. The last edition, the fifth, was printed in 1835. The next work was his essays, literary, moral, and philosophical, published contemporaneously with the Medical Inquiries. Rush died in this city in 1813, at the age of sixty-eight. The slanders which were heaped upon him were a disgrace to his age and country. To such an extent were these slanders carried by Cobbett, the editor of a scurrilous paper called the Porcupine, that Rush, at the earnest solicitations of his friends, instituted against him a suit for libel, the jury awarding him $5000 damages, every cent of which he distributed among the poor of Philadelphia. Cobbett, driven into bankruptcy, and treated with contempt by his fellow-citizens, soon after went to New York, where for a short time he edited a new paper, named the "Rushlight," in which he continued his abuse of the illustrious physician. The latter days of Rush were spent in comparative tranquillity in the retirement of his study, in the love and esteem of a large circle of friends, in the contemplation of religion and philosophy, and in the supervision of American editions of the works of Sydenham, Cleghorn, Pringle, and Hillary.

In connection with these splendid literary achievements of Rush, it is proper that I should pay a passing tribute of respect to a deserving man, a contemporary of the great physician, of whom the present generation of medical men is as ignorant as if he had never existed. I allude to Dr. John Jones, author of "Plain Remarks on Wounds and Fractures," the first edition of which was issued in 1775, and the last, namely, the third, considerably enlarged, in 1795, under the supervision of Dr. James Mease. The work comprises an interesting chapter on the construction of military hospitals, and an account of a case of hydrocele containing two gallons of fluid, one of the most extraordinary of the kind upon record.

Jones was a native of Jamaica, Long Island, of Welsh extraction, and a member of the religious Society of Friends. After having been for some time Professor of Surgery in New York, he removed to this city in 1780, where he became physician to Washington and Franklin, physician to the Pennsylvania Hospital, and vice-president of the Philadelphia College of Physicians. Much of his education was acquired under Pott and John Hunter. He is said to have been a very dexterous operator. His death occurred in the sixty-third year of his age.

Rush, as we have seen, died in 1813; and only two years before that event appeared Wistar's Anatomy, the first native systematic treatise on that subject ever published on this continent. In 1813 appeared Dorsey's celebrated Elements of Surgery, and soon after Chapman's Materia Medica and Therapeutics, all pioneer works, the result of the labors of professors in the University of Pennsylvania, then the foremost medical school in America. In order to carry out the plan I have proposed to myself, and to do full justice to the subject, it will be necessary to speak of the literature of each of the subdivisions of medicine, beginning with anatomy. Before doing so, however, I must be permitted to offer a few remarks respecting the textbooks in use in this country during the latter part of the last and the early part of the present century. It is proper to observe that during this period only three schools existed on this continent, the University of Pennsylvania, the New York College, and Harvard University. The text-books up to the close of the century must have been imported from England, which was itself but poorly supplied with medical works. The First Lines of the Practice of Physic, by the great Dr. William Cullen of Edinburgh, was published in 1776, and was the first scientific production of the kind in the English language. This celebrated treatise was reproduced in the latter part of the last century in the United States, and for a long time held its place as a text-book both in Great Britain and on this side of the Atlantic. An edition of it, with notes and observations, from the pen of the late Professor Charles Caldwell, appeared in this city in 1816. Of the character and value of these additions, the editor evidently had a most exalted opinion; for he declares, in pompous phrase, that the work without his notes is dangerous in its effects on the inexperienced cultivators of science, imbecile in its practice, and marked, in many cases, by unqualified error, "a fault that must necessarily have proved, in innumerable instances, signally mischievous in its influence on society." Alas! poor Yorick, if he could have risen from the dead, and found himself thus criticized, and that too by a man who never had a hundred patients in his life, what mental torture would he not have experienced! The whole secret of this denunciation was simply to promote the sale of Caldwell's Cullen, as it was called.

Another book, also unmercifully criticized by Caldwell, was The Modern Practice of Physic, by Dr. Robert Thomas, of Salisbury, England, issued in 1801. This he pronounced to be "a bloated and ill-digested compilation." Possibly, he may not have been alone in this opinion; but that all other physicians did not think so is sufficiently apparent from the fact that the Modern Practice of Physic passed through eleven editions in England, the last having been issued in 1853, in two volumes, and from the fact that it enjoyed for a long time a most extensive reputation in this country, having been edited, first, by Professor Edward Miller, and, after his death, by Professor David Hosack, of New York, both men of great eminence. An abridgment of the work, by Dr. William Currie and Dr. D. F. Condie, was issued in this city in 1817.

In physiology the only treatise extant at the time was that of Blumenbach, translated from the Latin by Dr. Caldwell in 1795. The most popular works on anatomy were those of Fyfe, and of the two Bells, John and Charles. The treatise on materia medica by Dr. Cullen was the text-book on that branch. Chemistry was little, if at all, studied in medical schools, and the only accessible works on that subject must have been those of Lavoisier, Fyfe, and Thomson. The works of Percivall Pott, of John Hunter, and of the two Bells, Benjamin and John, were the principal treatises on surgery. Smellie's midwifery was the only one on that subject in England during the latter part of the last century, to which was added, early in the present, the celebrated work, "The Principles of Midwifery," of Dr. John Burns, of Glasgow, the tenth edition of which was published in 1843, and which for upwards of a quarter of a century exerted a powerful and wide-spread influence upon the obstetric practice of this country.

2. ANATOMY AND PHYSIOLOGY.

To Dr. Caspar Wistar, Professor of Anatomy in the University of Pennsylvania, we are, as already stated, indebted for the first native work on anatomy ever published on this continent. It was issued in two parts in 1811, and in 1814 in two octavo volumes, under the title of "A System of Anatomy" for the use of students of medicine, and before it had reached its third edition its lamented author had ceased to live. Subsequently the work was edited by the late Professor William E. Horner, and, at a still later period, by my colleague, Professor Joseph Pancoast, under whose careful and patient supervision it received large additions, in the form of illustrations and new matter, chiefly in the department of minute structure, a branch of anatomy then, in great degree, unknown both in this country and in Europe, the eminent commentator himself verifying almost every statement by careful and repeated personal examination of the microscopical character of the tissues. To such an extent were these researches carried that, for a time, he suffered severely from morbid irritability of the eyes induced by over-exertion. When the work finally became obsolete as a text-book, after having enjoyed the confidence of the profession for a third of a century, it had passed through nine editions, denotive of an amount of popularity seldom attained by a scientific treatise. It does not appear to be generally known that the accounts of the bones, muscles, and ligaments, comprising nearly the whole of the first volume of the treatise, were verbatim extracts, respectively, from Monro, Innes, and Weitbrecht, upon those subjects. However this may be, the work was written with great clearness, and was, therefore, admirably adapted to the wants of the student. Wistar was the first to give an accurate description of the triangular extremities of the ethmoid bone, previously supposed to be portions of the sphenoid. Hence they have been known, ever since his death, in 1818, as the pyramids of Wistar.

After Wistar's treatise appeared, in 1826, that of Dr. William E. Horner, then adjunct and subsequently sole professor of anatomy in the University of Pennsylvania, a work in two volumes, entitled "Special Anatomy and Histology;" and then the elementary treatises of Morton, of Handy, of Richardson, and of Leidy, productions extensively employed as text-books, and composed, for the most part, by men of great reputation. The Atlas of Henry H. Smith and of Professor Horner, published towards the middle of the century, did good service in the cause of the anatomical student. No special notice need here be taken of those useful booklets, known as dissectors, of which Horner, Agnew, and Hodges have each furnished one. The Surgical Anatomy of the Arteries by Professor N. R. Smith, of Baltimore, deserves high commendation, inasmuch as it is a work of rare excellence, written by an able anatomist and surgeon, fully acquainted with the subjects he undertook to describe and discuss. The late Dr. Usher Parsons, of Rhode Island, for one year professor of midwifery in this College, early in life, published a valuable volume on anatomical preparations. Dr. John D. Goodman contributed a small brochure on the fasciæ, founded on personal dissections. Dr. John Neill is the author of a small work on the Anatomy of the Arteries, Nerves, Veins, and Lymphatics.

On Surgical Anatomy no complete separate treatise has yet appeared by an American author. In 1822, Dr. William Anderson, of New York, published Part I. of A System of Surgical Anatomy; and Drawings of the Anatomy of the Groin with Anatomical Remarks, by Dr. William Darrach, a folio volume, appeared in 1830.

Of William Edmonds Horner it is but little to say that he was one of the most accomplished anatomists of this or any other age; he was much more; he was a Christian gentleman, and an honest, upright man, the noblest work of God. Born in Virginia, in 1793, he received his degree of doctor of medicine in 1814, in the University of Pennsylvania, in which he gradually worked his way up from the office of prosector to Dr. Wistar through the demonstratorship and adjunct professorship of anatomy to the full professorship of anatomy, which he held up to the time of his death in 1853. During our late war with Great Britain he served with great credit as assistant surgeon, performing important duties both in the field and in the hospital. It was while making his hospital rounds one day, that he was accosted by an armless man with a constant titter on his face. "What's the matter? This does not strike me as a subject for laughter." "It is not, Doctor, but excuse me, I lost my arm in so funny a way that I still laugh whenever I look at it." "What way?" "Our first sergeant wanted to be shaved, and as I am corporal we walked out together in front of his tent. I had lathered him, taken him by the nose, and was just about applying the razor, when a cannon ball came, and that was the last I saw of his head and of my hand. Excuse me, Doctor, for laughing so. I never saw such a thing before." Dr. Horner was not a good writer nor a brilliant lecturer; but whatever he wrote, or whatever he uttered in the amphitheatre, bore the impress of truth and conscientiousness, seldom witnessed in any walk of life. As a minute anatomist and as an elegant dissector, he was probably never surpassed. Many of the most beautiful preparations in the Wistar and Horner Museum of the University of Pennsylvania are enduring monuments of his skill and patience as a great anatomist.

In General Anatomy the only native production is that of Professor Peaslee, of New York, published in 1857. Previously to its appearance, our knowledge of this branch of the science had been derived, mainly, from the works of Bichat, Beclard, and Bayle and Hollard, translated, respectively, by Hayward, Togno, and Gross. Dr. Tyson's Practical Histology, a small volume, was published a few years ago.

In pathological anatomy, the works of Horner, of Gross, and of Delafield are the only ones from the pens of American writers. The treatise of Horner, although abounding in useful knowledge, is devoid of scientific arrangement, and deficient in completeness. The morbid anatomy of Asiatic cholera is well described, and is illustrated by beautiful drawings, from the author's own dissections, made during the visitations of this frightful disease in 1832 and 1833 in this city. My work on pathological anatomy was issued in two volumes in 1839. It was composed while I held the chair of pathological anatomy in the medical department of the Cincinnati College, and was the first attempt ever made in the English language to systematize our knowledge upon the subject. It passed through three editions, in the preparation of the last of which, issued in 1857, I was assisted by my colleague, Dr. Da Costa. The second, however, I have always myself regarded as the best, as it connected an account of diagnosis with diseased structure, the only way in which, as I conceive, these two branches of medicine can be successfully studied. The Handbook of Post-mortem Examinations and of Morbid Anatomy of Dr. Francis Delafield, issued in 1872, is mainly intended, as the name indicates, as a guide to persons engaged in post-mortem dissections. This, with the exception of detached papers in our periodical literature, and the Transactions of the Pathological Societies of Philadelphia and New York, is all that has been done in this country to advance the interests of one of the most important departments of medicine that can engage the attention of the student, a branch which should be prominently taught in every well organized school.

The only contributions made to the study of comparative anatomy, in book form, are the lectures of the late Dr. Jeffries Wyman, of Boston, and the little volume of Dr. Harrison Allen, of this city, entitled "Outlines of Comparative Anatomy and Medical Zoology."

Prolific as the American press has of late years been, it has not yet furnished us with any original treatise on microscopical anatomy. That such a work, if based upon original investigations, would be well received does not admit of a doubt, and the time, I hope, is near at hand, when our young men will give the matter due attention. While upon this subject I may state that our Dutch brethren only a few weeks ago celebrated, at Delft, the second centenary anniversary of the discovery of microscopic animals by Leeuwenhoeck, a native of that town, and who was the first to direct attention to what is now a great science. What added to the interest of the occasion was the exhibition of the original instrument used by this great man in his examinations.

If we turn to Physiology we shall find in our literature an abundance of material, worthy of any age or country. Commencing with the Human Physiology of Dunglison, we have the work of Martyn Paine, of wide scope and much erudition; of Dr. Draper, author of the immortal treatise on the Intellectual Development of Europe; of the admirable elementary treatise of John C. Dalton, the universal text-book of our schools, written in the purest and clearest English; and, lastly, the elaborate and exhaustive treatise of the younger Flint, in five volumes, upon the composition of which not less than twelve years of precious labor were consumed. Well written and elaborately treated, it is without a rival in the English language, and is destined to exercise a salutary influence upon the progress of physiology in the United States. I need say nothing here in the way of commendation of the work of the late Dr. Oliver, of Boston, or of the Institutes of Medicine of the late Dr. Gallup, of Vermont. The Human Physiology of Dr. Robley Dunglison, issued in two volumes, in 1832, has, in my opinion, not been equalled in erudition and scholarship since the days of Haller. Like the work of that illustrious physiologist, it is a lasting monument to the genius and industry of its author, a work which, although no longer used as a text-book, will be consulted in all time to come by the inquisitive student, as a bright mirror reflecting, thoroughly and completely, the history of physiology, as it was understood and taught throughout the world, during a period of a quarter of a century. Long before the death of its lamented author, in 1869, it had reached its eighth edition.

The Treatise on Human Physiology, by Professor Draper, is a great production, although it is now obsolete as a text-book in the medical schools. Being a profound chemist as well as a most able physiologist and physician, the author has discussed many of the functions of the body in a manner and with a degree of skill rarely found in works of this description. The treatise has been honored with a translation into the Russian language.

Under this head may be mentioned the remarkable treatise of Dr. James Rush, of Philadelphia, the "Philosophy of the Human Voice," issued in 1827; a work which has passed through six editions, the last having appeared in 1867, and which contains, as is asserted by competent critics, "a more minute and satisfactory analysis of the subject than is to be found in any other work."

3. CHEMISTRY.

Chemistry cannot boast much of its literary career on this continent. Its systematic works are few, and, with several exceptions, of no special credit as national productions. Dr. Franklin Bache, of Philadelphia, and Dr. John Gorham, of Boston, took the lead in this particular branch of American medical authorship, the "System of Chemistry" of the former, and the "Elements of Chemical Science" of the latter, in two volumes, having appeared almost simultaneously in 1819. The work of Dr. Bache was especially designed for the use of students of medicine. Dr. John White Webster, professor of chemistry in Harvard University, in 1825, published a manual of chemistry, which enjoyed some popularity in its day. This man, noted for his high culture and high position, social and professional, in 1849 perpetrated one of the most atrocious murders on record, his victim being Dr. George Parkman, a personal friend and estimable citizen. For this crime Webster was hanged in the yard of the Leverett Street jail, Boston, in 1850, after a full confession of the causes which led him to commit the act. Dr. James F. Dana, in 1825, published a small volume entitled "An Epitome of Chemical Philosophy," regarded as a very creditable performance at the time of its appearance. Dr. Robert Hare, professor of chemistry in the University of Pennsylvania, in 1828, furnished his class with a text-book, entitled a Compendium of Chemistry, chiefly valuable as a guide to his lectures. This gentleman, a native of Philadelphia, of English descent by the father's side, was, I have always thought, the most able practical chemist of his day in this country. He was a brilliant experimenter, but a dull, uninteresting lecturer; his great trouble being a want of power of expression before his class. When hardly twenty years of age he invented the oxyhydrogen blowpipe, a contrivance of great use in the investigation of chemical science, and which at once made his name widely known both in the United States and in Europe. He was a large contributor to the periodical literature of the time, and a man of capacious intellect, led astray ultimately by the phantom of spiritualism, the study of which engaged much of his attention during the latter years of his life. Dr. Hare died in 1858, at the age of seventy-eight years.

In 1830–31 appeared the "Elements of Chemistry," by Prof. B. Silliman, Sr., in two volumes; and about the same time the "Manual of Chemistry," by Lewis C. Beck, and the "Philosophy of Chemistry," by Dr. Thomas D. Mitchell, formerly a professor in this school. The latter work never passed into a second edition. Professor Silliman, Jr., published his "First Principles of Chemistry" in 1846; and in 1852 appeared the "Class-Book of Chemistry," by Professor E. L. Youmans; two works which have been largely used in our schools and colleges, and have had an immense circulation. Dr. John A. Porter is the author of "Principles of Chemistry," issued in 1856. Of the excellent "Manual of Medical Chemistry" of my colleague, Professor Rand, I need not here speak, as you are either already, or will soon become, familiar with its contents. It is a remarkable fact that the more elaborate works on this branch of science have been the productions of the pens of non-medical men.

What we need in this country, above all things in this branch of medicine, is a great work on organic chemistry, founded upon original observations made in the laboratory, patiently and steadily conducted through a series of years, not written in a day by pilfering other men's thoughts. Who, among you, will undertake it?

Under the present head may be mentioned the great work of the late Dr. Samuel L. Metcalfe, formerly Professor of Chemistry in Transylvania University, Kentucky, on "Caloric; its Mechanical, Chemical, and Vital Agencies in the Phenomena of Nature," issued, in two volumes, in 1843, and again in 1853; a production of great labor, of extensive research, and of deep thought. The publication of this work, effected under many difficulties, placed its author among the foremost philosophers of the age. It was particularly well received abroad; and it is asserted that it induced a wish, on the part of the trustees of the University of Edinburgh, that Dr. Metcalfe should become a candidate for the then vacant Gregorian chair in that celebrated institution. Dr. Metcalfe was a native of Virginia, and died in 1856, having spent many years abroad.

Although our systematic literature in chemistry is very meagre, volumes upon volumes of detached papers, upon almost every conceivable subject, are scattered through the periodical press, amply attesting the activity, talent, genius and researches of hosts of earnest workers in this grand and varied field of science. A large proportion of these papers, so creditable to the century, made their appearance originally in Silliman's American Journal of Science and Arts, that marvellous repository of mental labor, which has maintained its place in the confidence and esteem of the scientists of the whole civilized world for upwards of half a century. An enumeration even of the titles of the contributions of some of these chemists, as, for instance, those of Lawrence Smith and of Benjamin Silliman, Jr., would occupy many pages. It is a noteworthy fact that Dr. Benjamin Rush was the first professor of chemistry in America, having been elected to the chemical chair in the University of Pennsylvania in 1769. He had attended the lectures of Dr. Joseph Black, of Edinburgh, where he had no doubt become fully imbued with the importance of a knowledge of this branch of science as an aid to the medical practitioner. The great teacher has left no record of his chemical labors.

4. MATERIA MEDICA, THERAPEUTICS, AND BOTANY.

Our literature is opulent in works on materia medica and therapeutics, of which that of Dr. Nathaniel Chapman, of this city, the earliest of all, was issued, in two volumes, in 1817–19. Eberle's treatise, also in two volumes, appeared in 1822; and after that, in more or less rapid succession, the publications of William P. C. Barton, John B. Beck, Robley Dunglison, Martyn Paine, John P. Harrison, George B. Wood, Thomas D. Mitchell, William Tully, Alfred Stillé, John B. Biddle, and John C. Riley. The popularity of the works of Chapman and Eberle was very great, and that of the latter was accorded the honor of a German translation at Weimar soon after its appearance in this country. The great merit of Professor Stillé's elaborate and erudite treatise, issued in 1860, is attested by the numerous favorable criticisms pronounced upon it both by the American and European press, and by the fact that it is already in its fourth edition. Of Professor Biddle's excellent volume it will be sufficient to state that it is one of the favorite text-books of the medical schools of the United States. The learned works of Dunglison and of Wood enjoyed a wide reputation in their day.

Under the head of materia medica may be noticed the several dispensatories published in this country, works needful alike to the physician, the apothecary, the pharmacist, and the druggist. The first native production of this kind was from the pen of John Redman Coxe, of this city, issued in 1806, and such was its success that it passed through not less than seven editions. The American New Dispensatory, by Dr. James Thacher, of Barnstable, Massachusetts, appeared in 1810, and also met with marked favor, especially in New England. In speaking of Professor Coxe's work, Dr. Thacher observes: "The author of the American Dispensatory, printed at Philadelphia, has conferred an honor on the author of this work—the American New Dispensatory—by transferring literally from the two last editions more than forty pages into the fourth edition of his own without the customary quotation marks or marginal references." Such wholesale plagiarism would have afforded fine material for a spicy paragraph in the "Calamities of Authors" by the elder Disraeli. "If," says the author of the Anatomy of Melancholy, "the severe doom of Synasius be true, that 'it is a greater offence to steal dead men's labor than their clothes,' what shall become of most writers?" To steal the labor of the living is not a less crime! It is worthy of notice that Dr. Coxe, who was evidently an accomplished chemist, in 1816, published a paper in Thomson's Annals of Philosophy, entitled "A Plan for Electric Telegraphy," long antedating, as stated by Professor Silliman, Jr., any other American suggestion on this subject since the days of Franklin.

The works of Coxe and of Thacher were superseded by the more able, scientific, and elaborate Dispensatory of George B. Wood and Franklin Bache, a great national production, the first edition of which appeared in 1833, and the last—the thirteenth—in 1875. Of the popularity of this book, the offspring of an accomplished physician and of an able chemist, an idea may be formed when it is stated that nearly 100,000 copies of it have been distributed during the period here specified. Professor Bache, the predecessor of Professor Rand in the chemical chair of this School, died in the spring of 1864, and thus the preparation of the last two editions was devolved upon the surviving author at a period of life when such labor, however agreeable or congenial in the vigor of manhood, must have been exceedingly irksome and exhausting. Associated together in the publication of the work, preparing edition after edition, often in rapid succession, an enterprise which brought these distinguished men almost into daily contact, it is gratifying to know that a friendship, begun upwards of half a century ago, was never marred by a single cloud, but burned with undiminished lustre down to the hour of Dr. Bache's demise. It is also gratifying to know that Dr. Wood, at a ripe old age, is still among us, full of honor, a crown of glory to his profession, and an ornament to his age and country. When he shall be gathered to his fathers, it will be fit that a garland, woven by the hands of the medical and pharmaceutical professions, of both of which they were such distinguished members, should be placed upon the tombs of the authors of the United States Dispensatory.

The Pharmacopœia of the United States owes its origin to the Massachusetts Medical Society, which, in 1808, appointed Dr. James Jackson and Dr. John C. Warren a committee to prepare such a work in conformity with the modern chemical nomenclature, in order to establish uniformity in the prescriptions of physicians. The work was afterwards adopted by the Medical Society of New Hampshire, and made the basis of Thacher's Dispensatory. Since then it has assumed, under the name of the United States Pharmacopœia, a strictly national character, and is subjected regularly every ten years to a most thorough revision by a joint committee of physicians and pharmacists, appointed, respectively, by the American Medical Association and by the American Pharmaceutical Society.

As appropriate appendixes to the above publications may be mentioned the formularies of Ellis, Griffith, and Green, works of great merit in their way, not less than twelve editions of the first having been issued from the press. Parrish's Pharmacy, a great treatise, also deserves passing notice; so likewise does the once popular book on "New Remedies," a laborious and comprehensive compilation by Professor Robley Dunglison, widely circulated in its day, not less than six editions having been consumed.

In therapeutics, apart from materia medica, our stock is a slender one. In 1828, Dr. John Esten Cooke, Professor of Medicine in Transylvania University, published a treatise on Pathology and Therapeutics in two volumes, evincing great learning and research, but so thoroughly tinctured with the author's peculiar ideas of the theory and practice of medicine, that it never met with much favor from the profession. Dunglison published a treatise on Therapeutics in 1836, which was subsequently issued under the title of Materia Medica and Therapeutics. A valuable essay on Infant Therapeutics was furnished by the pen of the late Dr. John B. Beck of New York. In 1867, Professor S. Henry Dickson published a small volume, entitled "Studies in Pathology and Therapeutics" The latest production upon this subject is the excellent work of Dr. Horatio C. Wood, the only one, I believe, in the English language which treats fully of the physiological action of drugs.

A considerable number of works on Botany, from the pens of medical men, have appeared in this country. Of these, the earliest perhaps was that of Professor Benjamin Smith Barton, published in 1803, and followed, in 1817, by the American Medical Botany of Professor Jacob Bigelow of Boston, in 3 volumes octavo, and, a few years later, by the magnificently illustrated Flora of North America, by William P. C. Barton, U. S. N., for several years professor of botany and materia medica in this school. The works of Dr. John Torrey, of New York, of Dr. William Darlington, of West Chester, Pennsylvania, and of Dr. Lewis C. Beck, of Albany, New York, are well known throughout the country. A treatise on medical botany, the latest of which was published in 1847, by Dr. Griffith of this city, is much needed to bring up our knowledge to a level with the existing state of the science. Of these various writers the most copious is the late Professor John Torrey, a native of New York, and for many years Professor of Chemistry and Botany in the College of Physicians and Surgeons of that city. His contributions comprise a number of volumes, several of them beautifully illustrated. In 1860, Dr. Torrey presented his extensive botanical library and his magnificent herbarium, the fruit of the labor of forty years, to Columbia College, New York.

5. PRACTICE OF MEDICINE.

When I entered upon the study of medicine, in 1825, the works on anatomy, mainly, in use among teachers and students, as text-books, were those of Wistar, Fyfe, John and Charles Bell, and the Edinburgh System, as it was called. General anatomy was little, if at all cultivated; and the only treatise upon the subject was that of Bichat, translated a short time previously by the late Dr. George Hayward, of Boston. Microscopical anatomy, now so much cultivated, had no existence. On pathological anatomy, the only work accessible to the American student was that of Dr. Mathew Baillie, of London, a mere record of individual experience, "void and without form," although not without value in its day.

My text-book on surgery was that of Dorsey, which I read with much care, and thought it a great work, not, perhaps, without reason, considering the period at which it was written. On my arrival in Philadelphia, I obtained a copy of Sir Astley Cooper's Lectures on Surgery, edited by Tyrrell, a work which did much to shape the character of my mind, and to inspire me with love for this branch of the healing art. It was not a great work, but it was full of interest, and written in the plainest possible language. My fondness for it still lingers in my breast. Subsequently I read the writings of Pott, of Desault, of Abernethy, and of Samuel Cooper, a military surgeon, and later in life Professor of Surgery in the London University. His first Lines of Surgery, issued at London, in 1807, was long used both in Europe and in this country as a text-book in the schools, and his Dictionary of Surgery, published originally in 1809, and recently reproduced by Mr. Lane, of London, in a greatly improved form, is an imperishable monument to its author's memory, unrivalled, as the production of one man, for its accuracy, learning, and research.

The text-books on physiology were those of Magendie, Richerand, and Bostock; on materia medica and therapeutics, Chapman and Eberle; on chemistry, Turner, Hare, and Henry; on medicine, Cullen, Thomas, and Thacher; on midwifery, Burns, with notes by Professor James of the University of Pennsylvania; on medical jurisprudence, Beck. The only medical dictionary in use at the time was that of Hooper, soon afterwards superseded by the great work of Dunglison. Up to this time we had few national works; but they now began to multiply, and soon assumed an imposing character. Among the foremost writers of this period were Eberle, Dewées, Wood and Bache, Wood, and others. I look upon the Practice of Medicine of Eberle, issued in 1831, as forming an era in the medical literature of this country. It appeared in two volumes, and passed through not less than five editions during the author's lifetime, another having been issued after his death, with notes and additions by his friend and former colleague, the late Professor George McClellan. The work was long used as a text-book in our schools, was written in a lucid, classical style, and filled a void in our medical literature, universally felt at the time of its publication.

Almost simultaneously with the admirable work of Eberle, appeared that of Dr. W. P. Dewees, entitled "A Practice of Physic," in two volumes, the author being at the time Adjunct Professor of Midwifery in the University of Pennsylvania. He had previously issued his very able work on Obstetric Medicine, a work so far in advance of his Practice of Physic that his friends always deeply regretted the publication of the latter treatise, which, I believe, never reached a second edition. Although it contained much that was really valuable, the style was detestable. A reviewer in the North American Medical and Surgical Journal, in commenting upon the subject, fitly remarks: "Addison and Johnson have been little imitated in its pages; we must take the work as we find it; be thankful; and, with honest Sancho, exclaim, God bless the giver." The very best article in the book—the only one unexceptionably written—was the chapter on diseases of the eye by Dr. Isaac Hays.

In 1832, Dr. Samuel Jackson, Professor of the Institutes of Medicine in the University of Pennsylvania, published a volume entitled the "Principles of Medicine," a work so thoroughly tinctured with the doctrines of Broussaism that, although it sold rapidly, it completely disappointed the expectations of the profession. It is of this work that Caldwell wrote so scorching a review that the author, one of the most accomplished gentlemen and popular teachers of his day, would never issue another edition.

In 1842, Professor Dunglison favored the profession with a treatise on the Practice of Medicine, in two volumes, extensively used as a text-book by the students of this College, in which the illustrious author was so long a professor. The work, written in the elegant and lucid style for which he was so justly distinguished, reached its third and last edition in 1848, six years after the first.

Sixteen years had elapsed since the appearance of the treatises of Eberle and Dewees, when the great work of Dr. George B. Wood, at the time Professor of Materia Medica in the University of Pennsylvania, was ushered into existence. Issued in two portly volumes, written with great care and finish, characterized by a lucid, elegant, and scholarly style, systematic in the arrangement of its subjects, and exhaustive in its scope, it at once addressed itself to the good sense of the profession, and speedily became the leading text-book of the schools. Many copies of it found their way into Great Britain. Edition after edition, each succeeding one a great improvement upon the preceding, appeared, until 1866, when the sixth and last was issued. As a faithful embodiment of the art and science of medicine of the middle of the present century, the treatise of Dr. Wood cannot be too highly estimated. I know of no contemporaneous work upon the same subject, in any language, at all equal to it.

The Elements of Medicine by Dr. S. Henry Dickson, the first edition of which was issued in 1855, while the author was a resident of Charleston, is a work of great merit; but, from some cause or other, was never fully appreciated by the profession. The second and last edition appeared in 1859. To those who are familiar with the character of Dr. Dickson, with his accomplishments as a scholar, and with his ability as a writer, it is hardly necessary to say that the work is marked by that ease and grace of style so characteristic of that distinguished medical philosopher. The memory of this good and great man will long be held in affectionate remembrance by the many pupils who listened to his prelections during his connection with this School, delivered in a manner so peculiar, so graceful, and so scholarly, as to charm every one within their reach.

The work of Dr. Austin Flint must speak for itself. Having from an early period of his life been a public teacher, a hospital physician, and a close observer of disease, it is not surprising that he should have produced a work of matchless ability, far in advance, in point of diagnostic and nosographic accuracy, of any treatise of equal bulk in the English language. A sufficient evidence of its popularity, and of the estimate placed upon it, is the fact that it is already in its fourth edition, the first having been struck off in 1866. I regard it as by far the most original treatise on the principles and practice of medicine ever published in this country, an opinion in which I am supported by the entire profession.

The Essentials of the Principles and Practice of Medicine, by Professor Henry Hartshorne, is a work of great popularity, well and concisely written, a fourth edition having lately appeared within a short period of the original issue. It is emphatically a handy-book for students and practitioners.

Professor N. S. Davis, of Chicago, several years ago, published a volume on Clinical Medicine, which recently passed to a second edition. As a record of the experience of the distinguished author, running through a period of forty years, in a large private and hospital practice, the book possesses no ordinary value.

I must not omit to mention in this connection that a volume on the practice of medicine by Dr. David Hosack, of New York, for many years a professor of medicine in that city, one of the deepest thinkers and best writers of his day, was issued after his death, by his early friend, Dr. Ducachet. Of the merits of this work I am unable to judge; but of this I am positively certain, that, at the date of its publication, it was far in arrear of the existing state of the art and science of medicine. In 1824, about ten years before his death, which was caused by apoplexy induced by losses sustained in the great fire in New York, which laid waste much of his property, Dr. Hosack published three volumes of "Essays on Various Subjects of Medical Science," exhibiting not only a thorough knowledge of the subjects treated of, but an ease of style and an elegance of diction rarely met with in medical authorship. As a finished scholar, a polished gentleman, a graceful writer, an astute practitioner, and a man of genius, few physicians have ever surpassed him.

Under the present head may be included a brief notice of the American Cyclopædia of Practical Medicine and Surgery, edited by Dr. Isaac Hays, begun in 1834, and suspended at the end of the second volume for the want of adequate encouragement. It contains many able and learned articles from the pens of different writers, especially those of Dr. Geddings, at the time Professor of Anatomy in the University of Maryland, on Amputations and on the Arteries; on Aneurism, by Dr. Hugh L. Hodge; on the Anus, by Dr. Reynell Coates; and on Asphyxia, by Robley Dunglison. It was designed to give the work a national character, and one's only regret is that it was not pushed forward to completion.

Of medical monographs on the disorders of particular organs or regions, the number is by no means inconsiderable. Thus, on the Thoracic Organs—the heart and lungs—may be mentioned the excellent treatises of W. W. Gerhard, John Swett, N. Chapman, Lawson, Austin Flint, Loomis, S. George Morton, René La Roche, and Meredith Clymer; on Croup, John Ware; on the Diseases of the Throat and Larnyx, J. Solis Cohen and Antoine Ruppaner; on Fever, Thomas Miner, Nathan Smith, N. Chapman, John K. Mitchell, Caspar Morris, Elisha Bartlett, René La Roche, Meredith Clymer, and J. E. Reeves; on Nervous Affections, Oliver Wendell Holmes, Brown-Séquard, and William A. Hammond; on Delirium Tremens, John Ware; on Nature in Disease, Jacob Bigelow; on Cerebro-spinal Meningitis, Alfred Stillé; on Urinary Deposits, Frick, Flint, Jr., Tyson, and Fowler; on Epidemics, Joseph Mather Smith; on Hypodermic Medication, R. Bartholow; on Medical Diagnosis, J. Da Costa; on Pain, S. H. Dickson; on Cutaneous Maladies, Worcester; on Erysipelas, Minor; on Thermometry, Seguin; on Apoplexy and Cerebral Hemorrhage, Lidell.

In the group of works here enumerated are several which deserve special commendation. In point of originality those of Brown-Séquard on nervous affections hold the first rank. The discourse on Self-Limited Diseases by Bigelow, published in 1835, opened a new mine both of doctrine and of practice. The treatises of Gerhard and of Austin Flint are models of their kind, based as both are upon thorough personal observation. The estimate attached to the Medical Diagnosis of Da Costa is attested by the fact that, although issued only in 1864, it is already in its fourth edition. The treatise of Bartlett, the History, Diagnosis, and Treatment of Typhoid and Typhus Fever, issued in 1842 while the author was Professor of Medicine in

Transylvania University, is founded chiefly upon the labors and researches of Louis, Chomel, and Andral among the French, and of Nathan Smith, Jackson, and Hale of New England.

As a work of profound erudition, at once complete and exhaustive, written in a scholarly style, and evincing the most patient and extraordinary research, the monograph on Yellow Fever, by Dr. La Roche, is without a rival in any language. The author was at great pains and expense in obtaining everything that had been written upon the subject, and, as he himself expresses it, neglected no opportunity of rendering himself practically familiar with the disease of which he thus became the distinguished historian. The facts borrowed from the numerous writers consulted by him seem to have been verified in every instance by personal reference to their works, a task in itself of immense labor, enough, indeed, to cause the eye and brain to ache and the hand to tremble. We talk of the writings of Scott, of Cooper, of Irving, and of Dickens as something extraordinary, if not gigantic, and so in truth they are; but here is a work of which even few professional men have ever heard, and of which the public is wholly ignorant, which caused its accomplished author an amount of brain labor far greater than any ever experienced by these great men, who are worshipped almost as demigods. One page of the treatise of La Roche on yellow fever, one of the great scourges of the human race in tropical climates, embodies more toil, more close thinking, more accurate statement of facts, than any chapter of fiction that has ever been written. The work is a model of its kind, reflecting the highest credit upon our national literature.

Several valuable Manuals, as they are called, intended to facilitate the labors of the medical student during his attendance upon lectures, have been published by Mr. Lea, and have enjoyed a wide circulation. Their authors, John Neill and Francis G. Smith, Henry Hartshorne, and J. L. Ludlow, are well known Philadelphia teachers and practitioners. A work by the late Dr. Mendenhall, of Cincinnati, was constructed upon a similar plan.

A very curious work, not without interest and instruction, was published, in two volumes, in 1858, by Dr. L. M. Knapp, formerly Professor of Midwifery in Rush Medical College,

Chicago, entitled "Researches on Primary Pathology and the Origin and Laws of Epidemics." The object of Dr. Knapp is to prove that all diseases are caused by a scorbutic diathesis: and so thoroughly is he convinced of his success that, in announcing his discovery, he adopts the enthusiastic language of Kepler in his Harmonices Mundi: "Eighteen months ago I saw the first ray of light; three months since I saw the day; a few days ago I saw the sun himself, of most admirable beauty. Nothing can restrain me; I yield to the sacred frenzy." "Time," says Dr. Knapp, "is the arbiter of all things;" "all great truths," he complacently adds, "have first to be announced." Although seventeen years have elapsed since the world was first apprised of these wonderful revelations, I question whether there is a solitary physician who has become a convert to them. The work of Dr. Knapp fell stillborn from the press, the victim, apparently, of the scorbutic diathesis.

It is very difficult in a discourse like this to assign a just position to the great work of Dr. Daniel Drake, for many years my colleague and warm personal friend, one of the great luminaries of the profession, and the pioneer physician of the West. Of the nature and vast scope of this work, its comprehensive title is a sufficient indication—"A Systematic Treatise, Historical, Etiological, and Practical, on the Principal Diseases of the Interior Valley of North America, as they appear in the Caucasian, African, Indian, and Esquimaux Varieties of its Population." The first volume was issued in 1850, and the second in 1854, two years after the death of the lamented author, under the joint supervision of Dr. Hanbury Smith, of Ohio, and Professor F. Gurney Smith, of this city. Drake had long contemplated writing such a work; but it was not until a comparatively late period of his life that he found leisure to collect the necessary materials. For this purpose long and tedious journeys were undertaken attended with great fatigue, heavy expense, and great sacrifice of practice. Like Rush, Drake had many irons in the fire, which, in more respects than one, were constantly kept in an incandescent state. His first tour was performed in the summer of 1837, during which he spent three months in the South, accompanied by his two daughters, the cherished objects of his home after the death of Mrs. Drake.

In 1843 he visited Alabama, Mississippi, Louisiana, Florida, and the Gulf of Mexico, and, subsequently, Tennessee, Kentucky, North and South Carolina, Virginia, Western Pennsylvania, New York, Indiana, Illinois, Michigan, Iowa, Wisconsin, Missouri, Canada, and the great Lakes. Much of the material thus collected was arranged for the press during the lecture terms of the University of Louisville, where, in a little room on the second floor, this great medical philosopher used to lodge and breakfast, his other meals being generally taken promiscuously among his many friends who always welcomed him with a cordial greeting. If the work of Drake did not fall stillborn from the press, it has been so coldly received by the profession that it has never passed into a second edition. As it was unsuited for a text-book it could not be used by the student, and to men in active practice it was less convenient as a book of reference than the treatises of Eberle, Wood, Watson, Bennett, and others. The style was strongly Anglo-Saxon, like everything Drake ever wrote, and the arrangement of its topics was admirable. The materials of which it was composed were collected, for the most part, by personal intercourse with the physicians of the States and Territories which he visited for the purpose, a novel mode, seldom practised, of acquiring information. The whole profession of the interior valley of North America was thus laid under contribution. I consider the work a great performance, and I am sure that future ages will agree with me in my estimate of its high value.

Of Medical Dictionaries may be mentioned those of Dunglison and of Joseph Thomas, the former of which, without a rival in the English, if, indeed, in any language, has stood its ground, as a work of reference, for forty years, the first edition having been issued at Boston in 1833, and the last, or sixteenth, thoroughly revised and enlarged, in 1874, under the supervision of Dr. Richard J. Dunglison, a son of the illustrious author.

6. SURGICAL LITERATURE.

In his surgical studies, prior to the early part of the present century, the American student relied solely for his knowledge upon the reprints of foreign works. In native productions, of late so numerous, and, I may add, so creditable to the country, Dr. John Syng Dorsey, the nephew of Physick, and Adjunct Professor of Surgery in the University of Pennsylvania, led the way. His Elements of Surgery, comprised in two octavo volumes, was issued in 1813. Written in a style remarkable for its simplicity and clearness, it was designed for the use of students, but must also have been of great service to the profession generally, so much in need at the time of an exponent of American views and practice. Laying no claims to originality, it was a mere epitome of the science, largely made up of extracts from the treatises of contemporaneous authors, such as Desault, Boyer, and Benjamin and John Bell, interspersed with an account of the opinions and experiences of American surgeons, especially those of Physick, whose teachings were everywhere regarded as dicta from which there was no appeal. The work was illustrated by engravings, not very creditable to the fine arts even in those days, but, nevertheless, very graphic and valuable. A portion of the preface of the Elements is so remarkable in its bearings upon the then surgical practice of England and France, that I shall not hesitate to present it here. "An American," says the author, "although he must labor under many disadvantages in the production of an elementary treatise, is in one respect better qualified for it than a European surgeon. He is—at least he ought to be—strictly impartial, and therefore adopts from all nations their respective improvements. Great Britain and France have been foremost in the cultivation of modern surgery, but their deficiency in philosophical courtesy and candor has in some instances greatly retarded its progress. To illustrate this remark it will be sufficient to state that the doctrine of adhesion, so ably developed in England, has been shamefully neglected in France; and that French surgery in fractures finds no advocates in Britain. Some of the best writings of Desault have never been translated into the English language, and those of Hunter are unknown or disregarded throughout the continent of Europe. This spirit of hostile rivalship, extending from the field of battle to that of science, cannot fail to exert a pernicious influence on practical surgery; a truth too palpable to escape the observation of any foreigner who visits a European hospital.

An American, in walking their wards, sees with surprise in London a fractured thigh rudely bound in bundles of straw, and the patient discharged limping with a crooked limb. In the French capital he witnesses an amputation, and is disgusted by the officious zeal with which the surgeon crams a handful of lint between the stump and the flap which covers it, with an express design to prevent their adhesion. It is difficult to reconcile these facts with one equally true, that, among the most distinguished men who have ever adorned the profession of surgery, are living characters in London and Paris." Since these lines were penned, upwards of sixty years ago, a new order of things has arisen, and the two nations here referred to in such disparaging terms, readily appropriate each other's labors in whatever is good, or calculated to promote their common welfare.

Dorsey died in 1818, soon after the publication of the second edition of his unpretending volumes. A third edition was issued in 1823, and another at a still later period, with notes and additions, by Dr. John Randolph. The work was highly appreciated in this country, and it is worthy of notice that it was used for many years as a text-book in the University of Edinburgh, for a long time the foremost school of medicine in Great Britain, if not in the world.

The treatise of Dorsey was succeeded by the Institutes and Practice of Surgery, by Dr. William Gibson, also a professor in the University of Pennsylvania, the first volume having appeared in 1824, and the second in 1825. In its original form the work was inexpressibly meagre, if not contemptible—utterly unworthy of the high position occupied by its author, introduced into the school as the successor of Physick. Altogether it passed through eight editions, and, as each one was a marked improvement upon its predecessor, the work at length assumed a very respectable character, in striking contrast with the parent imprint. Among its greatest merits was the remarkable clearness of its style.

Of the Principles and Practice of Surgery of the late Dr. George McClellan, my old master, the founder of this college, a brilliant lecturer, an expert operator, and a man of rare genius, it would not become me to speak. It was an incomplete production, hastily written, and should never, in my opinion, have been published. It was issued from the press in 1848, a short time after the death of the lamented author, under the supervision of his son, the late Dr. John H. B. McClellan. Decidedly the best part of the volume is that which is taken up with the narration of cases, which, although not always accurate, nevertheless displays remarkable vigor and great descriptive power, indicative of a master spirit, and reminding one forcibly of the graphic style of John Bell, of Edinburgh. A curious circumstance connected with this work is, that the preface was written long before any portion of the body of the work. McClellan was descended from a Scotch family, and was born at Woodstock, Connecticut, in 1796. He obtained the charter for this college in 1825, and was its Professor of Surgery until 1838. His death occurred after a brief and sudden illness, in 1847, in the fifty-first year of his age.

In 1859 appeared the work of S. D. Gross, followed in rapid succession by that of Henry H. Smith, of John Ashhurst, and of Frank H. Hamilton; treatises the bare mention of which must suffice for my present purpose.

The works of Professor Geddings, of Charleston, South Carolina, and of Dr. John Hastings, U. S. N., require no special notice. The former was intended as an outline of the course of lectures annually delivered by its distinguished author, and the latter as a brief resumé of the art and science of surgery as it existed a quarter of a century ago. Neither of these works has reached a second edition.

Such, then, is our stock of systematic treatises; quite enough, if properly posted from time to time, for the next fifty years. The literature of operative surgery has been illustrated by the labors of the elder Pancoast, and, more recently, by those of Dr. Henry H. Smith and Dr. John Packard. The first edition of Professor Pancoast's splendid work, a work which has achieved for him a world-wide reputation, was issued in 1844, and the last—the third—in 1852. It is comprised in a quarto volume, illustrated by eighty lithographic plates, interspersed through the text, many being from original drawings, and all of them executed in the highest style of the art. It exhibited, at the time of its publication, a complete view of the various operative procedures, preceded, in every instance, by admirable outline sketches of the surgical anatomy of the structures interested, and was by far the most complete treatise on operative surgery in the English, if not, indeed, in any language. Of the labor bestowed upon the preparation of the work by its illustrious author, it is unnecessary to speak; it is a monument of industry and of talent, and will indissolubly associate the name of Joseph Pancoast with American medical literature and the progress of American surgery. It is much to be regretted that the author, still in the full vigor of health and life, cannot be induced to prepare a new edition of the work, enriched by his vast personal experience, and brought up fully to the level of the existing state of the science. Such a performance, for which he is so well qualified, would be an invaluable legacy to our school and its numerous alumni, as well as to the profession at large, a profession which he has so much illustrated and adorned.

Dr. Henry H. Smith, in 1852, published a System of Operative Surgery, and four years afterwards a treatise on Practical Surgery, which, in 1863, were incorporated in one common treatise in two volumes, under the title of the Principles and Practice of Surgery. The work is beautifully illustrated, and is particularly valuable on account of its literary and historical references. Packard's Handbook of Operative Surgery is also handsomely illustrated, and is distinguished by great clearness of style. The Handbook of Surgical Operations, by Stephen Smith, issued in 1863, was of great service to our army surgeons during the late war, and has been deservedly well received. It is already in its fifth edition.

In 1857 Professor Paul F. Eve published a "Collection of Remarkable Cases in Surgery," forming an interesting and instructive volume, the matter of which is generally given in the language of the respective reporters, with occasional comments by the distinguished editor. As a book of reference, it possesses great value, exhibiting, as it does, on the one hand, the blunders in diagnosis and practice of eminent surgeons and physicians, and, on the other, the wonderful recoveries that not unfrequently occur after injuries and operations, apparently under the most adverse circumstances.

Of books on minor surgery, the only native ones, so far as my information extends, are those of Henry H. Smith, Fitz-william Sargent, John H. Packard, and Philip S. Wales, U. S. N., the latter being the most complete treatise on the subject ever published.

The revolutionary war was barren of results in regard to the literature of Military Surgery. Although the army was well supplied with physicians and surgeons, many of them men of professional mark in their day, the only publications of any importance emanating from them were the papers of Dr. Benjamin Rush and of Dr. James Tilton, on the diseases and management of military hospitals; that of the former being afterwards included in his collected works, Medical Observations and Inquiries, already alluded to. Both these gentlemen occupied high official positions during the war of independence. The tract of Dr. Tilton was written, in part, in 1781, at a time of general reform in the army, and received the approbation of a committee of Congress, of which Robert Morris was chairman. It was subsequently much enlarged, and issued in 1813 under the title of "Economical Observations on Military Hospitals and the Prevention and Cure of Diseases incident to an Army." For an opportunity of examining this little volume, now exceedingly scarce, I am indebted to my friend, Dr. W. Kent Gilbert.

Dr. Tilton, the author of this work, was no ordinary man. A native of Delaware, he served with great distinction during the continental war, rendering himself particularly conspicuous as a director of hospitals, into the economy of which he introduced most important improvements, thereby saving many lives. Towards the close of the war, he was elected Professor of Surgery in the University of Pennsylvania, but declined the honor; was present at the surrender of Lord Cornwallis at Yorktown, and, when the army was finally disbanded, he returned to Delaware, and resumed the practice of his profession. At the outbreak of the late war, as it is called, between this country and Great Britain, in 1812, he was appointed physician and surgeon-general to the army of the United States, and again distinguished himself by his services both in the field and in the hospital. The last days of this great and good man were spent in retirement at Bellevue, near Wilmington, where he expired in 1822, at the close of his 77th year.

Among the principal contributors to military medical and surgical literature during our war with England are Dr. James Mann, of New York, whose work, entitled "Medical Sketches of the Campaigns of 1812, '13, and '14," issued at Dedham, Massachusetts, in 1816, is replete in interest; Dr. Usher Parsons, of Providence, Rhode Island; and Dr. W. E. Horner, of this city. The observations of the last two, collected during their term of service, have not been published in book form.

In 1808, Dr. Edward Cutbush, U. S. N., published a volume of observations on the means of preserving the health of soldiers and sailors; and, in 1817, appeared the treatise of Professor William P. C. Barton, U. S. N., on the internal organization and government of marine hospitals; two works which accomplished much good in their day. A small volume on Diseases and Injuries of Seamen, by Dr. G. R. B. Horner, U.S.N., was issued in 1854; Hints on Recruits, by Dr. Thomas Henderson, U. S. A., in 1856, and the Manual of the Medical Officer of the Army, by Charles S. Tripler, in 1868.

The list of works on military surgery published during our late war, is quite formidable, although the works themselves are comparatively slender, most of them having been written to meet an approaching emergency felt by our surgeons. The Hand-book of Blackman and Tripler and the Manual of Gross appeared almost simultaneously, and received a warm welcome. Of my own booklet several thousand copies were disposed of during the war, and I have now on my table a copy of a translation of it into the Japanese language, accompanied by a letter from our Minister at Tokei, and one from the Surgeon-General of the Japanese army, informing me of the rapid progress which the Japanese people are making in the civilization of the western nations. Mr. Bingham declares that the American and European physicians, resident in Japan, have done more towards this enterprise than any other class of men. Professor Hamilton's treatise, published in 1865, is a more comprehensive production than either of the above works, and embodies much valuable matter, gleaned from personal experience. The "Manual of Military Surgery" of Dr. J. Julian

Chisholm, issued in 1861, at Columbia, South Carolina, was the text-book of the Confederate military surgeon during the late war, and is a work of superior merit, comprised in a duodecimo volume of 529 pages, profusely illustrated, and interspersed with brief details of interesting cases. It had passed, within three years of its publication, into a third edition. The treatise has everywhere received high commendation, especially from foreign critics. All these productions, however, excellent as they are, are thrown into the shade by the Medical and Surgical History of the War, authorized by Congress in 1869, and issued under the supervision of Dr. Barnes, Surgeon-General U. S. Army. The work, which is to consist of three parts, the first of which, comprised in two costly and magnificently illustrated quarto volumes, one on medicine, edited by Dr. J. J. Woodward, and the other on surgery, edited by Dr. George A. Otis, with an elaborate appendix, the joint labor of these two gentlemen, has been for some time published and widely distributed. Part II. is in process of preparation, nearly one thousand pages of it being already in print. When completed, the work will be an honor to the national government, and reflect imperishable credit upon Surgeon-General Barnes and his able assistants.

In connection with this subject I must not omit to mention, in terms of praise justly due, Dr. William A. Hammond's Military Medical and Surgical Essays, prepared in 1864, for the United States Sanitary Commission; and the Surgical Memoirs of the War of the Rebellion, collected and published by the same association. Only two volumes, edited by Professor F. H. Hamilton, have thus far been issued; but they comprise articles of great and enduring value, based upon personal observations in the field and hospital, interspersed with the results of the experience of the military surgeons of this and other countries. Professor Hammond has written an excellent treatise on military hygiene; and Dr. Joseph J. Woodward, U. S. A., has contributed an able work on the "Chief Camp Diseases of the United States Armies as observed during the War."

Orthopædic, plastic, and conservative surgery have received valuable contributions from the pens of Mütter, H. H. Bigelow

Sayre, Bauer, Taylor, Davis, Prince, Walter, Knight, and others. The surgical affections of the anus and rectum have been illustrated by Bushe and Van Buren; tumors, by John C. Warren; wounds of the intestines, by S. D. Gross; congenital dislocations of the hip, by J. Murray Carnochan; inflammation, by A. H. Stevens and John Packard; dislocations of the hip, by John C. Warren; fractures and dislocations of the hip, by Prof. Henry H. Bigelow; ophthalmic surgery, by Frick, Littell, Williams, and J. M. Gibson; aural surgery, by Turnbull and Roosa; fractures and dislocations, in an incomparable and exhaustive treatise, by Frank H. Hamilton; the treatment of fractures of the lower extremities, by N. R. Smith; the diseases and injuries of the urinary organs, by Parrish, Gross, Morland, and Gouley; the genito-urinary organs, by Van Buren and Keyes; spermatorrhœa, by Bartholow; excision of the joints, by Hodges; spinal disorders, by Taylor, Ashhurst, and Lee; pelvic surgery, by Sims, Bozeman, Agnew, and Emmett; surgical affections of the air-passages, by Green, Gross, J. Solis Cohen, Elsberg, and others; injuries of the nerves, by S. Weir Mitchell; diseases of the bones, by J. Nott and T. M. Markoe; earth dressing, by A. Hewson; optical defects, by C. S. Fenner. I may add that my treatise on the Diseases and Injuries of the Bones and Joints, issued in 1830, contains the first account of adhesive plaster as a surgical appliance in the treatment of fractures.

On Syphilis, the treatise of Bumstead, repeatedly reprinted at home, and translated into several foreign languages, occupies a prominent position in this variety of our literature. The work of Dr. Durkee, upon the same subject, is also a very creditable one, well received by the profession. In 1864, Dr. William A. Hammond published an able little volume on venereal diseases. The treatise of the late Dr. William W. Sanger, of New York, entitled "The History of Prostitution," is an exhaustive and meritorious production. The work, issued in 1859, and long out of print, deserves to be reproduced with such additions, of course, as have been made to the literature of the subject since the date of its publication.

Valuable contributions to surgery, of a miscellaneous nature, are to be found in Professor N. R. Smith's Medical and Surgical Memoirs, comprising an account of the observations of some of the writings of his distinguished father, Nathan Smith, of New Haven; in the Surgical Reports of George Hayward, in the Surgical Observations of the late lamented J. Mason Warren, and in the Contributions to Practical Surgery, by the late Dr. George W. Norris.

7. OBSTETRIC MEDICINE AND DISEASES OF WOMEN AND CHILDREN.

Obstetric medicine may justly boast of a number of works, which enjoy not only an American but European reputation. Dr. Samuel Bard, a professor in the Medical College of New York, is entitled to the credit of having been the first physician in this country to write upon the subject, his little treatise having appeared in 1807, in a duodecimo volume of 239 pages, under the title of "Compend of the Theory and Practice of Midwifery." Being entirely elementary in its scope, and without any pretensions to originality or claim to a scientific character, its chief design was to aid midwives and young practitioners in the exercise of their vocation. The author, after a career of great usefulness, beloved by all who knew him, a great favorite with the ladies, died at an advanced age in 1821. It is reported of Dr. Bard that he always took special care of his hands, which, in cold weather, he invariably carried in a fur muff, both in walking and in riding, in order to preserve the delicacy of their touch as well as their beauty.

The man who imparted the first real impulse to our obstetric literature, and who elevated its practice to the highest rank, was Dr. William P. Dewees, at first adjunct-professor and then sole professor of midwifery in the University of Pennsylvania. He was the prince of obstetric practitioners in this country. No lady in Philadelphia was considered as safe or fashionable if she was not attended in her accouchement by Dewees. He delivered, it is affirmed, at least ten thousand women during the active period of his professional life. He was the first on this continent to render midwifery truly respectable as an art and as a science. From his authority there was no appeal. By his writings and his teaching he rendered himself famous, both at home and abroad. Dewees was at once a dogmatist and a merciless critic. He cut right and left, fore and aft, sparing neither friend nor foe, native or foreigner. Everybody swore by Dewees, and Dewees swore by himself. For a third of a century his reign was supreme and undisputed. America had a school of midwifery, the creation of Dewees, who was at the same time its autocrat and its preserver. His celebrated System of Midwifery, issued about 1824, had, in 1854, thirteen years after the author's death, reached its twelfth edition, an honor rarely, if ever, bestowed upon any similar work. The style of this treatise, like that of everything he ever wrote, was slovenly and highly inaccurate. This man, often called the Baudelocque of America, so illustrious in his day, and so much caressed by the citizens of Philadelphia, died in 1841, at the age of seventy-three, in a state of poverty and mental imbecility.

The work of Dewees was followed by those of Meigs, Bedford, Henry Miller, Hodge, Byford, and Elliot; treatises which reflect great credit upon their respective authors, and embellish our national medical literature. The work of Dr. Henry Miller was honored, soon after its publication, with a reprint in London. He was a keen critic, a bold, but judicious practitioner, and a clear writer, well acquainted with the subjects on which he exercised the powers of his pen. Of all these treatises that of the learned and excellent Dr. Hodge is, perhaps, the most elaborate and scholarly, as it certainly is the most elegant. Bedford was a dashing writer, and his book was a great favorite with the profession, especially with the pupils of the University of New York, in which he was long a popular teacher. An extraordinary charm pervades the work of "dear old Meigs;" and the treatise of Byford is valuable on account of its directness and strong common sense. In connection with obstetric literature may be mentioned an elaborate and instructive volume, published, in 1848, by Professor Walter Channing, of Boston, entitled a "Treatise on Etherization in Child-birth, illustrated by 581 cases."

Dewees, Meigs, Bedford, Hodge, Byford, and Thomas have produced admirable treatises on the diseases of women; and the diseases of children have been ably illustrated by the writings of Dewees, Eberle, Stewart, Condie, J. Lewis Smith, and of Meigs and Pepper. A perfect gem in its way is to be found in the Essays on Infant Therapeutics, by the late distinguished Dr. John B. Beck, for many years professor of materia medica and therapeutics in the College of Physicians and Surgeons of New York. Old as this little volume is, it can never become obsolete.

To Dr. J. Marion Sims belongs the honor of having been the first to write a work in the English language on uterine surgery. A treatise on the diseases and displacements of the uterus, under the title of Hysterology, was published in 1872, by Dr. E. N. Chapman. J. Randolph Peaslee and Washington L. Atlee have produced able treatises, respectively, on ovarian tumors and the diagnosis of ovarian diseases; and Professor Barker, of New York, has recently furnished us with a classical and learned monograph on the puerperal fevers, already translated into several of the continental languages of Europe. I should be unjust to my feelings if I did not allude here, in connection with the diseases treated of by Professor Barker, to the admirable brochure upon the same subject by Professor Oliver Wendell Holmes, of Boston. A more able, philosophical, and convincing pamphlet, or one more opportune, is not to be found in our literature. It was a terrible blow to the Philadelphia non-contagionists. Professor Meigs' treatise on Childbed Fevers appeared in 1854.

8. MEDICAL JURISPRUDENCE.

The pioneer writer on Medical Jurisprudence in the United States was Dr. Theodoric Romeyn Beck, whose treatise was issued, in 1823, in two octavo volumes, and was the first attempt ever made in the English language to systematize our knowledge upon the subject. Republished in London in 1825, with notes and emendations, by Dr. William Dunlop, it passed through four editions in England and six in this country during the lifetime of its distinguished author. After his death a new and thoroughly revised impression was brought out by Messrs. Lippincott & Co., of this city, under the supervision of the late Professor Gilman, of New York, assisted by an able corps of colaborators. A German translation of the work appeared at Weimar, in 1828. Having long been familiar with the character of Dr. Beck's treatise, from the fact that I was myself once a teacher of legal medicine, I have no hesitation in stating it as my conviction that it was, in its day, the most comprehensive, able, and erudite production on the subject of which it treats in any language, and that it constitutes a lasting monument to the genius, industry, judgment, and learning of its lamented author, who, born at Schenectady, New York, died at Albany, in 1855, at the age of sixty-four years, deeply regretted by all who were acquainted with his name and his great work. Abandoning the practice of medicine in early life, he accepted the office of principal of the Albany Academy, a celebrated seminary, over which he presided upwards of twenty-five years, lecturing in the mean time annually on materia medica in the Albany Medical College, and contributing copiously to the periodical press, especially the American Journal of the Medical Sciences. His taste for the study of medical jurisprudence manifested itself, it is said, during his pupilage, and gradually ripened into full maturity with increasing years. It is but justice to add that the chapters in this grand book on fœticide and infanticide were furnished by Dr. John B. Beck, a brother of the author, for many years Professor of Materia Medica and Therapeutics in the College of Physicians and Surgeons of New York. I may also add that the Beck family consisted of four brothers, three of whom were eminent physicians, and the other a distinguished member of the St. Louis bar.

The treatise on Medical Jurisprudence by Dr. Moreton Stillé and Francis Wharton, Esq., formerly a prominent member of the Philadelphia bar, issued in 1855, was a worthy successor to the great work of Dr. Beck; Dr. Stillé furnishing the chapters on the fœtus and newborn child, on sexual relations, on identity, and on the causes of death. The work is now in its third edition, in three volumes, numerous additions having become necessary by the progress of science, and is one of the most valuable contributions ever made to the medical literature of this country. Dr. Stillé was a facile writer, an earnest student, and an accomplished scholar. That such a man should have died in the prime of life, before he had completed his thirty-third year, in the midst of his useful and brilliant career, is deeply to be regretted. His demise was a great loss not only to the profession but to the country. "They whom the gods love die young." I must not forget to add that the later editions of this work have received important additions from the pen of Prof. Alfred Stillé, a brother of the lamented medical author.

Dr. Thomas Cooper, a chemist, a physician, and, at one time, a district judge of Pennsylvania, in 1819, edited certain tracts on Medical Jurisprudence, comprising the sterile monographs of Farr, Dease, Male, and Haslam, with a preface, notes, and a digest of the laws relating to insanity and nuisance. When this work, a sad representative of English legal medicine, was issued, Cooper was Professor of Chemistry and Mineralogy in the Literary Department of the University of Pennsylvania.

Dr. Stringham, of New York, Dr Charles Caldwell, then of this city, Dr. John W. Francis, of New York, and Walter Channing, of Boston, delivered lectures on Medical Jurisprudence early in the present century, and no doubt contributed, in a very material degree, along with the great work of Dr. Beck, to diffuse a taste for the study of this important branch of medical science, at present so much neglected in our schools.

The Medical Jurisprudence of Insanity by Dr. Isaac Ray is a work of great merit, which, originally issued in 1838, has passed through five editions at home, and has been honored with a reprint both in England and in Scotland. Dr. John J. Elwell, at one time a member of the profession, but now a practising lawyer at Cleveland, Ohio, in 1860 published a valuable treatise on the medical jurisprudence of malpractice and medical evidence, or the legal relations between physicians and patients; the only work of the kind, so far as my information extends, in the English language. A treatise constructed upon a somewhat similar plan, entitled the Jurisprudence of Medicine in its relation to the Law of Contracts, Torts, and Evidence, was published in 1869 by Dr. John Ordronaux, professor of law in Columbia College, New York. Dr. William A. Hammond, in 1873, favored the profession with a treatise on Insanity in its relation to Crime. The maxim of the late David Paul Brown, Esq., of this city, the eminent criminal advocate, "that a doctor who knows nothing of law, and a lawyer who knows nothing of medicine, are deficient in essential requisites of their respective professions," cannot be too often repeated.

The question of criminal abortion has been well discussed by the late Professor Hugh L. Hodge of this city, in a small brochure published several years before his death; and by Drs. Horatio R. Storer and F. F. Heard of Boston, in a duodecimo volume issued in 1868, under the title of "Criminal Abortion, its Nature, its Evidence, and its Law."

9. TOXICOLOGY.

In respect to our toxicological literature we may boast of its quality rather than of its quantity, which is certainly very limited. The masterly treatise of Professor T. G. Wormley, of Columbus, Ohio, the "Micro-Chemistry of Poisons," atones, as I conceive, in a very great degree, for what would otherwise be great, if not inexcusable, defects in this branch of the subject. Issued in 1867, it at once assumed a national character as a standard work, sought after alike by the physician and the lawyer. Founded upon original investigations, extending through a series of years of the most patient and pains-taking labor, it is not surprising that it should be a recognized authority in our courts of law in all cases of poisoning requiring medico-legal skill for their solution. I have no hesitation in saying that the treatise of Professor Wormley, when fully appreciated, will do as much to elevate the literary and scientific character of the United States as any work that has yet emanated from our press. Not the least interesting circumstance connected with the history of this great treatise is the fact that the beautiful engravings which serve to illustrate it are the handiwork of Mrs. Wormley. This noble woman, who took upon herself this laborious task, and executed it in so able and skilful a manner as to elicit the admiration of the scientists of America and Europe, has her worthy counterpart in the no less noble wife of Mr. Allibone, the learned compiler of the great dictionary of authors, a work of which she re-arranged and re-wrote nearly 20,000 pages of MS. for the compositor.

Professor Reese, of the University of Pennsylvania, in 1874, published a manual of toxicology, comprising a resumé of the principal facts of the science; a work well adapted to the use of students and junior practitioners, as well as members of the bar.

Dr. Julius T. Ducatel, while occupying the chair of chemistry in the University of Maryland, published a manual of toxicology, the only contribution which, so far as I can ascertain, he ever made to our literature; a circumstance the more to be regretted because he had been a favorite pupil of Brougniart, Brouchant, and Gay-Lussac, and must, therefore, have been well qualified to develop and illustrate chemical science.

10. HYGIENE, ELECTRICITY, YELLOW FEVER, AND CHOLERA.

Of works on hygiene, general and special, our stock is small. In this branch of medicine, as in physiology, Dr. Robley Dunglison took the lead, his "Elements of Hygiene" having been published in 1835. Dr. Samuel Forry, a very able writer and a most earnest and devoted student, in 1842, favored the profession with a valuable treatise on the "Climate of the United States, and its Endemic Influences," a volume embracing a great deal of interesting matter, condensed into the smallest possible compass. The following year he published a work on meteorology. During the late war, while in the occupancy of the office of Surgeon-general of the United States, Professor William A. Hammond contributed a treatise on military hygiene, the first work of the kind ever issued on this side of the Atlantic.

Upon Medical Electricity, or the uses of electricity in medical and surgical affections, numerous works have appeared in this country, chiefly within the last ten years, some of them, as that of the late Dr. Charles E. Morgan, of Beard and Rockwell, and of Garrat, of an elaborate and exhaustive character. Among the more modest and less pretending productions of this class may be mentioned the compendiums of Dr. A. McLane Hamilton, Dr. F. Lincoln, Dr. W. B. Neftel, and Dr. Prince of Illinois.

On Mental Hygiene works of greater or less merit have been supplied by Amariah Brigham, William Sweetzer, Joseph Mather Smith, and Isaac Ray. The celebrated treatise of the latter on the medical jurisprudence of insanity has already been referred to. Dr. Ray, in 1874, published a small volume on mental pathology, a work which, like everything that has emanated from his pen, is of great value. The influence of diseases on the intellectual and moral powers has been well discussed in a treatise on this subject by Joseph Mather Smith, issued in 1848. Dr. John M. Galt, of Virginia, many years ago favored the profession with a monograph on the nature and treatment of insanity. In 1866, Dr. Edward Seguin, of New York, published a volume on Idiocy and its Treatment by the Physiological Method. Many able contributions, none, however, I believe, in book form, on insanity, have been furnished by the pen of Dr. Edward Jarvis. An exhaustive paper, by the same writer, on the census of the insane of Massachusetts, was published nearly a quarter of a century ago, and attracted much attention both at home and abroad.

Upwards of fifty years ago a system of philosophy of the human mind, known as Phrenology, and founded on the physiology of the brain, began to attract the attention of the medical profession of this country, its originator having been Dr. Franz Joseph Gall, of Germany. Its first advocate among us was Dr. Caldwell, soon after his return from Europe in 1820; but, although he wrote and lectured upon it in the principal cities of the Union, it excited little notice until the visit of Spurzheim in 1822, followed, some years later, by that of Mr. George Combe, who modestly styled himself its apostle. For a number of years the country rung with the wonders of the so-called science, and as a consequence numerous papers were written upon it, as well as some tracts, especially by Caldwell and John Bell of this city. For the last twenty years the subject has been in the keeping chiefly of charlatans, who still practise upon the credulity of the public. In the hands of Caldwell and of some of its other once earnest advocates it was supplanted by Mesmerism, and this, in turn, by Spiritualism, delusions which, as is well known, have enslaved and turned some of the best minds of this country and of Europe. When a man of such splendid intellect as Robert Dale Owen is rendered insane by the disturbances caused by such folly, it becomes the man of sense to visit it with unmeasured condemnation; in fact, as a criminal offence against the State.

Our Yellow Fever literature, as might be supposed, is very extensive, but, apart from the great work of La Roche, it is mainly comprised in pamphlets and papers in medical journals. Most of these publications have emanated from the pens of our Southern brethren, beginning, if I mistake not, with those of Charleston, South Carolina, where this scourge has been so frequently endemic.

Our Cholera literature is also very abundant. The frightful visitations of this disease, especially that of 1832, '3, and '4, have brought into the field numerous writers, most of whom have given very accurate and graphic accounts of the symptomatology of the malady, although not a solitary one has succeeded in throwing any actual light upon its etiology and treatment. Among the foremost physicians who have thus busied themselves may be mentioned Jameson, Drake, Bell, Condie, Jackson, Paine, Warren, Stillé, and H. Hartshorne. To this list may now be added the name of Dr. Ely McClellan, U.S. A., who, with the aid of the Supervising Surgeon-General, Dr. John M. Woodworth, has drawn up a full and lucid report upon cholera as it appeared in different localities in this country in 1873. Not the least valuable part of the work is an appendix by Dr. John S. Billings, U.S. A., comprising a complete catalogue of everything ever published upon this disease.

11. MEDICAL BIOGRAPHY AND MISCELLANEOUS SUBJECTS.

On general biography we have the works of James Thacher, in two volumes, issued in 1828; of Stephen W. Williams, in 1845; and of S. D. Gross, in 1861. That of the latter, entitled "Lives of Eminent American Physicians and Surgeons of the Nineteenth Century," embraces thirty-two sketches, contributed by twenty-nine writers. Dr. Toner, of Washington City, is the author of a brochure on general medical biography, comprising a kind of running commentary upon the lives of medical men who distinguished themselves during our colonial existence and during the revolutionary war; a most praiseworthy enterprise, requiring much research and patient examination, published in 1874 at the expense of the government. Of individual biographies, of which a number are before the profession, it would be useless on an occasion like this to speak.

A work of much historical interest, under the name of the "Writings of Hippocrates and Galen," was published in 1846 by Dr. John Redman Coxe, of this city, by whom it was epitomized from the original Latin translations. The work, comprised in an octavo volume of moderate size, is one of great labor and research, and forms a valuable addition to our medical literature. Dr. Coxe was one of the ablest Greek and Latin scholars that our country has ever produced, and he had the most extensive collection of the writings of the fathers of medicine in the United States, if not in the world. I may here add that Dr. Coxe, several years before his death, published an elaborate treatise to show that Harvey was not the discoverer of the circulation of the blood; a treatise which met with much ridicule and much caustic criticism, and convinced no one.

Honorable mention should be made here of the "Medical Profession of Ancient Times," a small volume, by the late Dr. John Watson, of New York, a classical scholar, thoroughly acquainted with the history of medicine. Dr. N. S. Davis, of Chicago, is the author of a History of the American Medical Association, edited by the late Dr. S. W. Butler, for many years editor of the Philadelphia Medical and Surgical Reporter. Those who are acquainted with the history of medical progress in this country need not be told that Professor Davis enjoys the high honor of being the originator of the American Medical Association. Dr. Robley Dunglison is the author of a History of Medicine, a posthumous production, edited by his son, Dr. R. J. Dunglison. The work of the late Dr. Worthington Hooker, of New Haven, "Physician and Patient," is a production of sterling merit, written by a man who fully understood the various subjects of which he treats, and which he has portrayed in a masterly manner. A Discourse on the Soul and on Instinct, by Martyn Paine, of New York, Essays on Life, Sleep, and Pain, by Samuel Henry Dickson, Sleep and its Diseases, by William A. Hammond, are booklets which admirably discuss these various topics, so replete in interest to the medical philosopher and the casuist. Letters addressed to a Young Physician, by the late Dr. James Jackson, of Boston, in two duodecimo volumes, published a few years before the death of that great and good man, are worthy of attentive study, embracing as they do many practical suggestions, based on the observations, experience, and reflection of half a century of medical practice. The letters are dedicated to Dr. John C. Warren, the author's life-long friend.

In the same category of works I must place that of the late Dr. R. D. Mussey on "Health, its Friends and its Foes," Boston, 1862, every word of which deserves to be read and re-read, on account of its valuable information. It is proper, however, to observe that the author was a great vegetarian, and that he occasionally, in his peculiar ideas, "oversteps the bounds of modesty."

Two works of a highly interesting character, well calculated to reward the labor of an attentive study, were published by the late Dr. Elisha Bartlett, a chaste and classical writer, and for many years an eminent teacher, one entitled the Philosophy of Medicine, and the other an Inquiry into the Certainty of Medicine. A careful perusal of the latter of these productions will serve to convince the reader that the distinguished author, if not a complete sceptic, had little faith in the efficacy of remedial agents. He believed that there was as much virtue in a dose of Rochelle salt as in one of calomel, and that rheumatism could be as readily relieved by the use of lemonade as of colchicum. As a teacher and as a writer Bartlett always reminded me of Dr. S. Henry Dickson; both had been my colleagues, both were elegant and polished scholars, both were good talkers and beautiful lecturers, both had poetic minds, and both were men of the highest professional and moral tone. The death of such men, so gifted and so rare, was a great loss to us.

The subject of Medical Education has been ably discussed, in distinct monographs, by Daniel Drake, John Ware, Robley Dunglison, and Samuel Chew. That of Drake, entitled "Essays on Medical Education and the Medical Profession in the United States," appeared in 1832. This was followed in 1847 by the Discourses on Medical Education and on the Medical Profession, by John Ware, of Boston. The Medical Student, or Aids to the Study of Medicine, by Robley Dunglison, was issued in 1837. The most recent publication upon the subject was from the pen of Dr. Samuel Chew, late professor of medicine in the University of Maryland, in "A Course of Lectures on the Proper Method of Studying Medicine."

Last of all, but not least, except in bulk, is the "Code of Ethics," adopted in 1847 by the American Medical Association, and since then by all the respectable medical societies of the United States, for the regulation of the conduct of physicians towards each other and towards the public; a booklet which, although the tiniest of all referred to in this discourse, is, nevertheless, worth its weight not in gold but in hundred-dollar greenbacks. Based upon the Medical Ethics of Dr. Thomas Percival, published at Manchester, England, in 1803, it owes its existence to a committee of the American Medical Association, of which Dr. Isaac Hays and the late Dr. Gouverneur Emerson, of this city, were prominent members, and to whom, as I have reason to believe, the code is mainly indebted for its present perfection. A booklet so precious and so useful, one calculated to prevent strife and to promote harmony and good feeling among medical men, should be the daily companion of the medical practitioner. I cannot recommend it too highly to your consideration. It is one of the great legacies of the age.

12. TRANSLATIONS AND REPRINTS.

There are two classes of men in our profession who are deserving of passing notice in connection with our medical literature on account of the part they have taken in making us familiar with the writings of European authors. I allude to the translators and editors, a very useful body of men, to some of whom it is impossible to award too much praise. Among the former, as, indeed, if I am not in error, among the latter, Dr. Charles Caldwell, a name famous in medical history, led the way, in association with Blumenbach's Physiology and Cullen's Practice of Medicine, celebrated works, long used as text-books in our schools. Of Irish descent, and born in a log cabin, in Caswell County, North Carolina, in 1772, the "young rustic" studied medicine in this city, where he soon became enamored with the prelections of Rush, and shortly after receiving his degree, "set up for himself," engaging in private teaching, often, like John

Brown, of Edinburgh, in opposition to the doctrines of his illustrious master. Commencing his literary career at an early period of his life, he busied himself in translating and editing foreign medical works, and in writing for Delaplain's Portfolio, a literary magazine, the first of any note in this country, established in 1812, under the editorship of Mr. Nicholas Biddle, the celebrated banker, whom he ere long succeeded in the management of the journal. Upon the organization of Transylvania University in 1819, at Lexington, Kentucky, Caldwell removed to that city, having accepted the chair of the Institutes of Medicine in that once famous school. Here he remained, in the enjoyment of a brilliant reputation, until 1837, when he assisted in founding the University of Louisville, his future theatre.

It will thus be seen that Caldwell was a pioneer, both as a writer and as a teacher. That he was a man of varied ability and remarkable attainment is sufficiently obvious. There was hardly any subject, professional or non-professional, which escaped his prolific pen. Indeed, he busied himself upon a greater variety of topics than any man our profession has ever produced. Altogether he wrote upwards of 10,000 pages of printed matter, embracing medicine, physiology, chemistry, ethnology, biography, phrenology, mesmerism, hygiene, insanity, sympathy, religion, temperance, the fine arts, gambling, oratory, language, and general education, which was one of his favorite themes. As a reviewer, he was always interesting, often caustic, and sometimes bitter and sarcastic, on special occasions sharpening his pen upon a brickbat, or dipping it into gall. His review of the work of the Rev. Samuel Stanhope Smith, President of Princeton College, on the causes of the variety of complexion and figure of the human species, was of so severe a character as to have occasioned, it is said, the death of its author from sheer chagrin, soon after its appearance. Another work, a strictly medical one, he handled so roughly as to induce the writer to recall the edition and consign it to the flames. He delighted in controversial writing.

If I am asked how Caldwell performed all his vast literary work, it will not be difficult to find an answer. He was all his life, an unusually long one, a bookworm. His mind was never distracted by practice, for he had none. He was, therefore, eminently a man of leisure; the master of his own time, and could thus devote himself, heart and soul, to the pleasures of his pen. As a teacher of physiology, which he expounded for upwards of a third of a century, I have no hesitation in saying that, when he retired from the University of Louisville, he was twenty-five years in arrear of the existing state of the science. Like Chapman, he was a solidist, unable to see any special use in the blood, except as a fertilizer of the system. As a writer, his style was diffuse, inflated, verbose, and, in the latter periods of his life, simply execrable. His dedication to Chapman, of his edition of Cullen's Practice of Medicine, was a fulsome and unmanly performance, beneath the dignity of a gentleman, dictated, as it was, by self-interest founded upon a promise that the work should be recommended as a text-book in the University of Pennsylvania, for a chair in which he was, for many years, an aspirant. His autobiography, published after his death, which occurred at Louisville, in 1853, at the age of 81, was composed in the worst possible taste, and is a libel upon most of the medical men with whom he was brought into contact. After all, he achieved no lasting fame as an author, although, as a mere writer, his name will always live. Had he confined himself to the production of a work upon some special subject, professional, scientific, literary, or philosophical, he might have earned immortal renown; as it was, he diluted his efforts by becoming, to use a common expression, a "Jack of all trades and master of none." If he had genius, and no one acquainted with him will deny him the possession of this gift, he expended it on too many subjects to become great in any one. Perhaps his very ablest production is his monograph on the "Original Unity of the Human Race," printed in 1851. It is questionable whether any publisher could be found at the present day to issue a select edition of his writings. To Caldwell must be accorded the title of Father of translators and editors of medical works. I may add that Caldwell was a gentleman of the old school; he had a splendid physique, a keen, penetrating black eye, and a large head, with the most courtly manners, and great colloquial powers. He had seen much of good society at home and abroad, could converse fluently and intelligently upon almost any subject that was presented to him, and was thoroughly a man of the world. I may also add that he was one of the vainest of men; and then, to complete the picture, I should add that he had something to be vain of.

To enumerate all, or to mention even a considerable number of the works which have been introduced in this manner into this country, would be a task as wearisome as unprofitable. I shall, therefore, select only a few of the more important ones. Among the earliest of the translations were Desault's Surgical Writings, by Edward Darrell Smith, of South Carolina; Larrey's Memoirs of Military Surgery, by R. Wilmott Hall; Bichat's immortal treatise on General Anatomy, by George Hayward, of Boston; Magendie's Physiology, by John Revere; the Surgical Works of Boyer, by Alex. H. Stevens; Broussais' History of Chronic Phlegmasiæ, by Isaac Hays and R. Eglesfeld Griffith; Tavernier's Operative Surgery, by S. D. Gross; Meckel's Anatomy, by A. Sidney Doane, of New York; Bertin's Treatise on Diseases of the Heart and Great Vessels, by Charles W. Chauncy; Beclard's General Anatomy, by Joseph Togno; Tanquerel on Lead Diseases, by Samuel L. Dana; Velpeau's Midwifery and Colombat on Females, by Charles D. Meigs; Velpeau's Surgical Anatomy, by John W. Stirling; and Velpeau's Operative Surgery, by R. S. Townsend, under the supervision of Dr. Valentine Mott, who has enriched its pages with a large amount of valuable matter, derived from the storehouse of his vast experience. More recently have appeared translations of Lehman's Manual of Chemical Physiology, by J. Cheston Morris; Cazeaux's Midwifery, by W. R. Bullock; Renouard's History of Medicine, by C. G. Comegys; Vidal's Treatise on Venereal Diseases, by George C. Blackman; Bernard and Huette's Operative Surgery, by W. H. Van Buren and C. E. Isaacs; Code of Health of the School of Salernum, by John Ordronaux; Stellwag's Treatise on Diseases of the Eye, by Roosa, Bull, and Hackley; Guersant's Surgical Diseases of Children, by Richard Dunglison; Billroth's General Surgical Pathology and Therapeutics, by Charles Hackley; Gluge's Pathological Histology, by Leidy; Malgaigne's Treatise on Fractures, by John H. Packard; Moritz Myers on Medical Electricity, by William A. Hammond; Rindfleisch's Text-Book of Pathological Anatomy, by William C. Kloman, assisted by Professor Miles, of the University of Maryland; and of Zeiss's Treatise on Venereal Diseases, by Frederick Sturges. At the present writing, Dr. Albert Buck, of New York, is engaged upon a translation of Ziemssen's Cyclopædia of the Practice of Medicine, in fifteen volumes, not less than four or five of the American edition having already appeared. Such an undertaking is denotive of energy and enterprise alike of the able editor and the public-spirited publishers.

Among the more useful and important foreign works reprinted in this country under the supervision of so-called editors, are the System of Surgery of Benjamin Bell, abridged by N. B. Waters, issued in 1791; Chaptal's Elements of Chemistry, by Dr. Woodhouse; Henry's Chemistry, by Benjamin Silliman; John Burns's Principles of Midwifery, by Thomas C. James; Thomson's System of Chemistry, by Thomas Cooper; Samuel Cooper's Dictionary of Surgery, first by J. Syng Dorsey, and then by Meredith Reese; John Bell's Principles of Surgery, abridged by J. Augustine Smith; Gregory's Elements of the Theory and Practice of Medicine, by Nathaniel Potter, of Baltimore, and Samuel Colhoun, of Philadelphia; Lawrence on Hernia, first by Joseph Parrish, and then by I. Hays; Good's Study of Medicine, by A. Sidney Doane; Turner's Chemistry, first by Jacob Green, and then by Robert Bridges; Elliotson's Principles and Practice of Medicine, by Thomas Stewardson; Hope on Diseases of the Heart, by C. W. Pennock; Stokes's Lectures on Medicine, by John Bell; Copland's Dictionary of Medicine, by Charles A. Lee; Tweedy's Medical Library, by W. W. Gerhard; Watson's Lectures, by Dr. D. Francis Condie, and then by H. Hartshorne; Mackintosh's Practice of Medicine, by Samuel G. Morton; Chelius's Surgery, by George W. Norris; Lawrence on Diseases of the Eye, by Isaac Hays; Forbes's Cyclopædia of Practical Medicine, by Dunglison; Pereira's Elements of Materia Medica, by Joseph Carson; Cooper's First Lines of Surgery, by Willard Parker; Liston's Practical Surgery, by Thomas D. Mütter; Liston's Elements of Surgery, by S. D. Gross; Quain's Human Anatomy, by Joseph Leidy; Quain's Anatomical Plates, by Joseph Pancoast; Erichsen's Surgery, first by Brinton, and then by Ashhurst; Carpenter's

Physiology, by Francis G. Smith; Churchill's Diseases of Women, by D. F. Condie; Cruveilhier's Anatomy, by Granville Sharp Pattison; Gray's Anatomy, by Richard Dunglison; Wilson's Anatomy, first by Paul B. Goddard, and then by William H. Gobrecht; Wharton Jones on Diseases of the Eye, by Isaac Hays; Ramsbotham's Midwifery, by W. V. Keating; Miller's Surgery, the Principles and Practice, by F. Sargent; Pirrie's Surgery, by John Neill; Wilde's Aural Surgery, by Addinell Hewson; T. Wharton Jones's Treatise on Defects of Sight and Hearing, by Lawrence Turnbull; Taylor's Medical Jurisprudence, by John J. Reese; Wells on the Eye, by I. M. Hays.

Some of the above works have been greatly improved by the notes and annotations of their respective editors—as, for instance, those of Cooper, Burns, Stokes, Watson, Graves, and Hope. When, in 1848, the Lectures of Dr. Stokes had passed through their third edition, such was the amount of matter furnished by Dr. Bell that he considered himself justified in affixing his name to the top of the title-page, his proportion of the work being upwards of 1400 pages; enough, in amount of material and variety of topics, to form a large separate volume. The value of Dr. Hope's treatise on Diseases of the Heart was greatly enhanced by the insertion of the results of the interesting and instructive experiments performed jointly by the editor, Dr. Pennock, and by his friend, Dr. Moore, of Rochester. Carpenter's Physiology received important additions from the pen of Professor Francis G. Smith. The late Professor Mütter greatly enhanced the value of Liston's Lectures on the Operations of Surgery by incorporating into them an abstract of his various surgical papers, originally contributed to the American Journal of the Medical Sciences and other periodicals. The additions are chiefly important in relation to plastic surgery, a subject to which the eminent editor had evidently paid much attention, and with which his name is so honorably associated both in this country and in Europe. Dr. Walter F. Atlee, of this city, in 1855, published a large volume on Clinical Surgery, from notes taken by him of Professor Nélaton's Lectures; a work of much value, as it illustrates the views and experience of one of the greatest surgeons of the age.

Of the influence which these translations and reprints have exerted in moulding the doctrines and practice of American physicians, it is, of course, impossible to form even an approximative estimate; that it has been very great, and, in the main, wholesome, the high character of most of the authors of them is, I am sure, a sufficient guarantee. Such works are usually selected with much care and judgment by the editors and publishers, and the sale of many of them has been very extensive as well as highly remunerative.

13. MEDICAL JOURNALS.

A vast amount of medical literature, such as it is, is comprised in what is known as medical journalism. The subject, indeed, is one of such magnitude as almost to preclude the possibility even of touching upon it on an occasion like this, and yet it is one which must not be wholly ignored. Many thousand volumes of this kind of literature are scattered through the libraries of this country, much of it unbound, if not uncut.

The first medical journal published in the United States was the New York Medical Repository, edited by Samuel Latham Mitchill, Edward Miller, and Elihu H. Smith, men of great celebrity in their day. It was begun in 1797, and continued for upwards of twenty years, often amidst great difficulties, as is generally the case with such enterprises. The Philadelphia Medical Journal made its appearance in 1804, under the supervision of Dr. Benjamin Smith Barton; and the year following the Philadelphia Medical Museum, edited by Dr. John Redman Coxe. The Philadelphia Eclectic Repertory started into existence in 1811. It was conducted by a society of physicians, and was suspended in 1820. This journal will always be famous from the fact that it contains the first account of Dr. Ephraim McDowell's operations of ovariotomy. In due time similar publications sprang up in Baltimore, Boston, Cincinnati, Lexington, Charleston, and, in fact, in almost every city of the Union. The Philadelphia Medical and Physical Journal, edited by Professor Nathaniel Chapman, one of the medical lions of his day, issued its first number in 1820, and, after a brilliant career, was succeeded, in 1828, by the American

Journal of the Medical Sciences, a periodical of world-wide reputation, edited anonymously until 1841, when the name of Dr. Isaac Hays appeared upon the title page, where it has remained ever since, lately in association with that of his son, Dr. I. Minis Hays. A periodical, the North American Medical and Surgical Journal, conducted by a galaxy of great men—Hugh L. Hodge, Charles D. Meigs, Benjamin H. Coates, Franklin Bache, and René La Roche—flourished in this city from 1826 until 1831, bequeathing us twelve volumes of great value. The Western Medical and Physical Journal, conducted by Daniel Drake and Guy Wright, of Cincinnati, and the Transylvania Journal of Medicine, under the management of John Esten Cooke and Charles W. Short, were ushered into existence in 1828, and struggled each through a period of about twelve years. The first number of the Boston Medical and Surgical Journal, now, like its Philadelphia compeer, venerable by its age and constancy, was issued in 1828. The New York Journal of Medicine and the Collateral Sciences, founded, and for some years edited, by the late Dr. Samuel Forry, had a long, and, in the main, a brilliant career, commencing in 1843, and ending in 1860. The Western Journal of Medicine and Surgery rendered good service under the able editorship of Drake, Yandell, and Colescott. The Nashville Journal of Medicine and Surgery, founded and edited by Dr. William K. Bowling, in 1851, assisted by Dr. Eve, has, by its wholesome criticism, exerted a most salutary influence over the profession of the southwest, especially of that of Tennessee, where, perhaps, greater attention is paid to the observance of our code of ethics than in any other State in the Union. Its veteran editor, upon retiring last spring, was succeeded by two gentlemen of ability, Professors Briggs and Summers. There is a curious history connected with the origin of this periodical kindly communicated to me by Professor Bowling, showing what a courageous, talented, and enterprising man may accomplish. A prospectus was issued in the summer of 1850, with a promise that the first number should appear in the following January. When the time arrived, but one subscriber had sent in his name, and he was a brother of the future editor. It was on this corner-stone that the work was founded.

The Chicago Medical Examiner, lately amalgamated with the Chicago Medical Journal, had a long and prosperous career under the enlightened editorial management of Professor N. S. Davis.

Most of these journals were issued quarterly, a few monthly, and only one of them, the Boston, weekly. The number of weeklies has of late years much increased, but at present there are only a few quarterlies, at the head of which stands the American Journal of the Medical Sciences, the ablest and one of the oldest periodicals in the world; a journal which has an unsullied record, is managed by a learned editor and an astute publisher, and bears upon its pages many of the most elaborate and erudite articles written on this side of the Atlantic. Its list of collaborators comprises the names of many of the most distinguished, learned, and earnest authors, teachers, and practitioners in the United States, and is a guarantee that the work, now in its forty-eighth year, is not likely soon to die. The country owes its venerable editor, Dr. Hays, and its talented and courageous publisher, a lasting debt of gratitude. The Journal is a library in itself.

Of the existing number of medical periodicals I am unable to afford any accurate information. It certainly cannot be much short of one hundred. Of the manner in which they are edited it is not a part of the design of this discourse to speak. That some of them are lean and destitute of vigor is undoubtedly true; but even the weakest may not be without some benefit to the profession in those regions of the country in which they are published. Nearly all are, it may be boldly affirmed, deficient in genuine criticism; and, on the other hand, it is equally certain that we rarely meet with an instance in which their pages are tainted by literary jaundice, or polluted by ribaldry and personality. The wholesome influence exerted upon some of these journals by the American Medical Editors' Association, lately instituted, is already apparent. It will not be out of place to add that many of these periodicals are con ducted by professors in the service of their respective schools; a circumstance greatly to be lamented, inasmuch as it must seriously affect the independence which should characterize such publications.

Much valuable matter is locked up in the transactions of our medical societies. The American Medical Association, now in the twenty-seventh year of its existence, has annually issued a volume, generally containing a very respectable amount of useful matter mixed up with no inconsiderable quantity of rubbish, not fit even for the pages of an ordinary medical journal. The Transactions of the New York State Medical Society, now embracing many volumes, are far in advance, in true spirit and scientific character, of any publications of the kind in this country. The meetings of the Society are always well attended, and its proceedings are conducted with uncommon vigor and intelligence.

14. MEDICAL THESES.

There is a species of medical literature peculiar to medical pupils, which, unfortunately, as I conceive, found its way into the New World from the Old, at the very commencement of the organization of our first medical school. I allude to what are called medical theses, or inaugural dissertations, the bug-bear of the student and the nuisance of the professor. Of this variety of medical literature our colleges have huge piles, especially the older and more popular ones; for every-spring, in the Ides of March, large additions are made to their archives, usually badly written, not unfrequently ungrammatical, generally devoid of scientific information, and of no use to anybody, for it is not too much to say that not one in fifty affords the slightest evidence of competency, proficiency or ability in the candidate for graduation. Often, indeed, they are not even composed by him; and occasionally, as I know from personal observation, they are plagiarized or copied, it may be verbatim, from such books as are within his reach, if not actually from the works of his preceptors. Happily, for the credit of the schools, few of these productions find their way into print. In the early history of medical teaching in this country the theses were generally written in Latin, as is still the case in some of the schools of Europe; and it was the custom, for a time at least, for the more prominent students to defend them publicly on commencement day. To answer the purpose for which they were originally designed, such papers should exhibit at least a respectable degree of scholarship, and be founded upon patient clinical observation or experimental researches, calculated to elicit new light and thus advance the interests of science and of the healing art. The best specimens of this kind of literature have been furnished by the French and German students, especially the former, many of whose theses occupy a high position in French literature, as is proved by the fact that they are often referred to in standard works. One of the first literary efforts of Dr. Charles Caldwell was the editing of two volumes of American theses, the productions chiefly of the earlier graduates of the University of Pennsylvania. It would be well if, on the birth-day of American independence, a bonfire could be made of this trash, as it exists, without exception, in all our medical schools; and it is devoutly to be wished that the regulation which prescribes the presentation of the inaugural dissertation were abolished. It is usually supposed that a Latin thesis is an evidence not only of superior talent and scholarship but even of genius; and hence the possessor of such gifts is generally the envy of his fellow-students, who regard him with feelings akin to those of the green-eyed monster. When I had the honor, in 1828, to receive my degree from this College, two of the candidates were in this position; their names were read out on commencement day, and, having been thus complimented, the natural conclusion was that they were destined to become distinguished members of the profession. The exercises being over they returned to their respective homes, one to Virginia, the other to Massachusetts, and from that day to this I have never heard anything of them. Their scholastic efforts had evidently produced a mental marasmus from the effects of which they never recovered. The dullest boy not unfrequently makes the brightest man.

15. WRITERS ON NATURAL HISTORY AND OTHER SUBJECTS.

It is worthy of note, in relation with the subjects of this address, that a vast amount of literary matter, highly creditable to the nation, and greatly promotive of the diffusion of useful knowledge among our people, not directly connected with medicine, has been furnished by physicians devoted to the study and cultivation of the natural sciences. Among the pioneers who thus distinguished themselves may be mentioned the name of Dr. Samuel Latham Mitchill, who was for a number of years professor of chemistry in one of the New York medical colleges, and who contributed many valuable articles on botany, mineralogy, and zoology to the periodical press during the first third of the present century. Many anecdotes, illustrative of the credulous and eccentric character of this man, who died in 1831, in the sixty-seventh year of his age, are extant, and might be recited here if time permitted. Dr. Parker Cleaveland, Professor of Chemistry at Bowdoin College, Maine, was the author of the first systematic treatise on mineralogy and geology ever published in the United States. It was issued at Boston in 1816, and was greatly instrumental in diffusing a taste for the study of those fascinating and useful sciences among our people. Dr. John D. Godman, a celebrated anatomist, linguist, and writer, who died at Germantown, in 1830, in the thirty-seventh year of his age, was the author of the first work on the natural history of quadrupeds ever published in this country. Dr. J. E. Holbrook, for many years professor of anatomy in the Medical College of the State of South Carolina, has rendered his name immortal by his great treatise on American Herpetology and his monograph on Southern Ichthyology. Everybody in this country is familiar with the name of Benjamin Silliman, fitly styled, during his lifetime, by Edward Everett, the Nestor of American Science. His great monument is the American Journal of Science and Arts, which he founded in 1811, and conducted with signal ability to within a short period of the close of his valuable and brilliant career. Dr. John C. Warren, the great New England surgeon, interested himself in the study of the mastodon and the fossil impressions in the sandstone rocks of the Connecticut River. The works of the late Dr. Josiah Nott, of Mobile, on the biblical and physical history of man, the types of mankind, and the indigenous races of the earth, works in some of which he was assisted by Gliddon, Samuel G. Morton, A. Maury, Pilszky, and J. Aitkin Meigs, are well known at home and abroad. The Crania Americana and Crania Ægyptiaca of Dr. S. G. Morton, a man of varied information, of great professional skill, an able anatomical teacher, and a classical writer, are productions which have made the name of their illustrious author a household word with the scientists of both hemispheres, and have added lustre to the scientific character of the age. In connection with ethnology I must not omit to allude, in terms of high commendation, to the lucid and learned papers of my colleague, Professor J. Aitkin Meigs, papers which have earned for him a wide reputation both at home and abroad; nor to those of the late Professor Jeffries Wyman, of Boston, a most zealous and accomplished scientist, naturalist, and comparative anatomist. Dr. Richard Harlan, in 1825, furnished his Fauna Americana, and in 1835 his Physical Researches. To our fellow-citizen, Dr. W. S. W. Ruschenberger, U. S. N., the country is indebted for a series of text-books on the natural sciences, which have been widely used in our colleges and higher seminaries of learning, and have been of great service in popularizing these studies among the different classes of our people. The names of DeKay, Rogers, Lewis C. Beck, Charles T. Jackson, the younger Silliman, and of many other medical men, are indelibly associated with the development of the natural history, geology, mineralogy, botany, and palæontology of a number of our States; and every intelligent person is familiar with the vast light that has recently been thrown upon these subjects in the far western regions of our country by Dr. Hayden and his assistants of the United States Geological and Geographical Surveys. The researches of Leidy have shed an imperishable lustre upon the country, and have caused him to be universally recognized as the American Owen. Rush, Caldwell, and Dunglison, not to mention others, performed a great deal of literary work outside of the profession. The Dictionary for the Blind, the joint labor of Dunglison and Chapin, was a great undertaking, comprised in three large volumes. Drake, at an early age, published his famous Picture of Cincinnati, a book which attracted crowds of immigrants to that city. Most of the manuals of chemistry, mineralogy, botany, and physiology used in our schools and colleges have been written by medical men, whose training has, for the most part, eminently qualified them for the task.

Among the members of our profession who have distinguished themselves as miscellaneous writers, or for their interest in, and genius for the liberal studies, may be mentioned the names of Dr. Charles Caldwell, for some years the editor of Delaplaine's Magazine; Dr. David Ramsay, an eminent practitioner of Charleston, South Carolina, and the author of a universal history in twelve volumes, a work celebrated in its day; John W. Francis, a man of wonderful intellect and accomplishments in general and art literature, a ready writer and a great wit; Dr. John W. Draper, author of the immortal work, the Intellectual Development of Europe, of a History of the War of the Rebellion, and of the Conflict between Science and Religion; and the Autocrat of the Breakfast Table, Dr. Oliver Wendell Holmes, anatomist, poet, novelist, magazine writer, and medical philosopher, a gentleman who, by a rare combination of talents and attainments, has shown that, if he had devoted himself exclusively to the culture and practice of his profession, he might have attained to the highest pinnacle of fame. The late Dr. Elisha Bartlett, for many years a prominent teacher of medicine, and a medical author of no mean ability, possessed a highly poetical mind, and wrote some beautiful verses, which go to prove that with more devotion to the Muses he might have achieved a reputation rivalling that of Mark Akenside or of Oliver Goldsmith, a man who, to use the language of Johnson, wrote like an angel, and talked like poor poll. Bartlett, a short time before his death, published a little volume of poems, entitled "Simple Sittings in verse for Portraits and Pictures from Mr. Dickens' Gallery." The late Dr. John K. Mitchell, for many years professor of medicine in this school, was the writer of two poems, one of them published as early as 1821. Among other papers which he contributed to the literary press was one entitled the "Wisdom, Goodness, and Power of God as illustrated in the Properties of Water." Dr. Jacob Bigelow, the Nestor of Medicine in New England, has produced many graceful and witty pieces of poetry, and is the reputed author of a *jeu d'esprit*, in imitation of several American writers, under the title of Eolopoesis. Dr. Robert Hare, the great chemist, it is said, occasionally indulged in poetical composition, and had a great fondness for the Muses. An elegant translation into English verse of the famous Code of

Health of the School of Salernum, highly creditable to the good taste and scholarship of the author, was published, in 1870, by Dr. John Ordronaux, of New York. This work, so full of curious and valuable knowledge, communicated in quaint but striking language, should occupy a prominent place in every well-selected medical library.

It is a significant fact that nearly all the great authors whose labors are commemorated in this discourse were, or are, teachers of medicine, or professors in medical schools. So far as my memory serves me, the only exceptions are Thacher, Condie, and La Roche, none of whom ever sat in a professor's chair. This fact goes to show that official position is a powerful incentive to authorship. A teacher, worthy of his position, must necessarily be a close student, and this very circumstance, by shaping his tastes and fitting him for the discharge of the duties of his chair, prepares him for the composition of works illustrative of the particular branch of science in which he is an instructor. The fame of most of the great schools of this and other countries is largely due to the number and character of the works supplied by their respective professors. Indeed, it may be assumed, as an established fact, that no institution of this kind can long sustain itself without the reputation thus acquired, however brilliant, able, or learned its corps of teachers as lecturers, practitioners, or scientific investigators. The University of Pennsylvania and the Jefferson Medical College, not to mention other schools, are largely indebted for their past and present prosperity to the fame of their authors.

Among the great thinkers of the medical authors of the century I unhesitatingly place in the highest rank, among the honored dead, Rush, Drake, and Caldwell; and, among the living, Martyn Paine and John W. Draper; as medical observers, W. W. Gerhard, the two Flints, John C. Dalton, J. M. Da Costa, T. G. Wormley, Brown-Séquard, W. A. Hammond, and S. W. Mitchell, not to mention others; as great and learned compilers, Robley Dunglison, René La Roche, Theoderic Romeyn Beck, Charles A. Lee, John Bell, Wood and Bache; as acute and caustic critics, William P. Dewees, Charles Caldwell, and John Watson; as elegant and exhaustive systematizers, George B. Wood, and René La Roche; as poets, or writers of a poetical mind, Elisha Bartlett, Jacob Bigelow, John K. Mitchell, S. Henry Dickson, and Oliver Wendell Holmes. The most copious authors are Dunglison, Caldwell, John Bell, Martyn Paine, and George B. Wood. The writers whose productions have enjoyed the widest circulation and been pecuniarily the most profitable to author and publisher, are Dunglison, Wood and Bache. Of the works of the former, at the time of his death, it is estimated that the sale had reached upwards of 125,000 copies, equal to between 150,000 and 160,000 volumes. Of the Medical Dictionary alone 55,000 copies had been issued. The circulation of the Dispensatory of the United States has also been enormous. The income from the works of these writers has been without a parallel in medical literature.

16. PIONEERS IN MEDICAL LITERATURE.

The authors who have led the way as pioneers in American medical literature are, Wistar in Anatomy, Dorsey in Surgery, Chapman and Eberle in Materia Medica and Therapeutics, Bache and Gorham in Chemistry, Eberle in Medicine, Dewees in Midwifery and the diseases of Women and Children, Beck in Medical Jurisprudence, Dunglison in Physiology and Lexicography, Wormley in Toxicology, and Brown-Séquard in Nervous Diseases.

Of these pioneers, nine are dead, leaving behind them names which will live in history, and which were warmly cherished by their contemporaries.

Caspar Wistar, who in point of time stands at the head of the list, was of German parentage, born in this city in 1761. He was a man of great dignity of character, of commanding presence, and fine colloquial powers, popular in the amphitheatre as an anatomical teacher, and distinguished for his social qualities and hospitable entertainments. It was his custom for many years after he rose to eminence every Saturday evening, during the winter season, to collect his friends around him, along with such strangers of note as might happen to be in the city. After his death in 1818, these gatherings were perpetuated, under the name of the "Wistar Parties," in honor of their founder, and it was only at the outbreak of the war that they were finally discontinued. No man could be a member of this club unless he was a member of the American Philosophical Society. It so happened that the last of these entertainments took place at my house in April, 1861.

John Syng Dorsey, a nephew and a pet of Physick, was one of the most popular men of his day, beloved by every one in and out of the profession, full of soul, a bon vivant, and a most acceptable lecturer, struck down, after a brief illness, at the age of thirty-five years, just as he was about to spring into the panoply of manhood as a great teacher and a brilliant surgeon. His last residence was in a large new house, at the southwest corner of Seventh and Walnut Streets, where now stands the commanding edifice of the Philadelphia Saving Fund Society. Here, as soon as he became quietly settled, he gave a jolly dinner to a number of choice friends, including the late Judge Peters, celebrated for his wit and humor. After the wine had been freely circulated, Mr. Peters went to the window, and calling the host to his side, said, loud enough of course to be heard by all the company, and pointing across Washington Square, once a Potter's field, to the penitentiary at the opposite corner, "Dorsey, you have a d—d poor prospect beyond the grave." In less than three weeks Dorsey was no more. His last illness was ushered in only a few hours after he had delivered a brilliant introductory to his course of lectures on anatomy in the University of Pennsylvania in 1818.

Nathaniel Chapman, the third on this honored list, was a native of Virginia, and, after his settlement in this city, rapidly rose to distinction, becoming a great favorite with his pupils and with the people of Philadelphia. Possessed of great bonhomie, of overflowing wit and humor, and of extraordinary colloquial powers, he was a great punster, the prince of physicians, and the idol of the social circle. As a teacher, he was uncommonly eloquent, notwithstanding the defects of his palate, which seriously impaired his articulation; and few men ever wielded a greater influence over their pupils than he did. His lectures were always enlivened by the recital of anecdotes, of which he had a large fund ready for any occasion. Chapman died in 1853, in the seventy-third year of his age.

Franklin Bache, whose System of Chemistry, as has been seen, appeared in 1819, was a great-grandson of Benjamin Franklin, and was born in this city in 1792. Receiving his medical degree at the age of twenty-two, he served with distinction, first as surgeon's mate and then as full surgeon in 1813–14 during the war with Great Britain, at the close of which he returned to Philadelphia, engaging in private practice, and entering upon that career as a chemical worker, teacher, and writer, which has so honorably and enduringly associated his name with the progress of our literature. In addition to the above treatise, Dr. Bache contributed many valuable papers to the periodical press, edited several foreign works on Chemistry, wrote a number of the articles in Hays's American Cyclopædia of Medicine and Surgery, and, in conjunction with Dr. George B. Wood, brought out the Dispensatory of the United States, furnishing the whole of the material relating to chemistry. On the re-organization of this College in 1841, he was appointed to the chair of Chemistry, which he worthily filled up to the time of his death in 1864. Dr. Bache was a man of varied information, an indefatigable student, and one of the most frank, kind-hearted, honorable men I have ever known.

Of John Gorham, who shares with Dr. Bache the honor of the pioneership in American chemical literature, I am unable to offer much information. His work, Elements of Chemical Science, was published, as we have seen, in two volumes, at Boston, in 1819, and was pronounced by the elder Silliman to be an able production. He was educated in the laboratory of Professor Hope of Edinburgh, and is said to have been an excellent instructor and a popular lecturer. He occupied the chair of chemistry at Harvard University from 1816 to 1827. He ended his brilliant career at an early age, mourned and regretted by all who knew him, as well as by the profession at large.

Under John Eberle I attended two courses of lectures on medicine in this school, and his name is attached to my diploma. He was a man of short stature, with a light olive complexion, a keen black eye, and a good forehead. He was a model of a student, reticent, patient, laborious, and brimful of his subject. Whatever he knew he knew well. As a practitioner he never ranked high, and as a lecturer he was not pleasing, although always instructive. Having no powers as a speaker, he always availed himself largely of the use of his MS. Poverty seems to have been his lot; it seized upon him early, and clung to him all his life. His days, it is said, were shortened by the inordinate use of opium and other stimulants. Of social qualities Eberle was wholly devoid. I never heard him laugh heartily in all my intercourse with him, which, during my residence at Cincinnati, was, for a time, frequent and familiar.

It will be interesting to you, as pupils of this school, to know that Eberle was its first Professor of Medicine, that he was a copious as well as a very learned writer, and that long before his death he enjoyed a national and European reputation. Not less interesting to you will it be to know that he was the son of poor parents, of German descent, that he was a most zealous student, and that, above all, he was the architect of his own fame and fortune. As one of his weaknesses, I may state that he was a firm believer in the powers of the divining rod. Dr. Eberle closed his earthly career at the early age of fifty years, in 1838, at Lexington, Kentucky, where he was at the time Professor of Medicine in Transylvania University.

Of William Potts Dewees I knew personally very little, the whole of my intercourse with him being limited to two occasions in which he met me in consultation in the case of a child laboring under convulsions. That he was a man of great prejudice not at all creditable to his exalted position, I have ample reason to know. As a lecturer on midwifery he was eminently instructive and entertaining; as a writer, unpolished and ungrammatical. His latter years were embittered by ill health and straitened circumstances.

Theodoric Romeyn Beck was a model of the Christian gentleman, amiable, modest, kind-hearted, considerate, charitable; a devoted father, and an exemplary husband. It is stated by his biographer, Dr. Frank H. Hamilton, that he composed the greater portion of the first edition of his work on Medical Jurisprudence while watching at the bedside of his beloved wife, during her last painfully protracted illness; a touching tribute to her virtues, and a beautiful exhibition of the kindness of his heart.

It is as if it were but yesterday that the voice, rich in melody and powerful in utterance, of the last of these honored dead resounded in our ears in this Hall, in which, during the last half of the century under review, nearly 7,000 young men, gathered from all sections of this continent, the West Indies, South America, Europe, and even the far East, have received a large share of the education which has fitted them for the discharge of the active duties of their profession. It was in this Hall that Dunglison taught for upwards of thirty years to admiring classes those principles of physiology, of hygiene, and of therapeutics which he knew so well how to impart; and it was in this Hall that he gained that wonderful ascendency over the minds of his pupils which a beloved and an honored preceptor alone can inspire. A profound scholar, and a man of vast learning, he was literally a walking encyclopædia. As a writer, he touched nothing that he did not adorn.

Of the two living pioneers in our medical literature, it is not my business to speak; it is gratifying to know that they are still among us, and that they are actively engaged in forwarding the interest of their respective pursuits, in which they have acquired so much fame.

17. REMUNERATION OF MEDICAL AUTHORS—LIFE OF BOOKS.

The compensation of medical authors is seldom flattering; but of this we should, perhaps, not complain, inasmuch as this is by no means peculiar to our profession, but is shared by nearly all literary persons. Besides, medical authors are seldom obliged to live in garrets, as is so often the case with poets, novelists, and magazine writers, for they generally rely upon their practice for their daily bread, and employ their pen altogether in a secondary manner. First editions, even of works of great value, rarely afford any compensation to their authors; it is only after the merits of a book are fully established that it becomes remunerative. I speak feelingly upon this point. The copyright of Eberle's treatise on materia medica, an eminently successful work in its day, was sold for two hundred dollars; and I do not think that the sale of the two bulky volumes of Drake, embodying the results of the labors of a whole lifetime, reimbursed him for one-tenth of the sum expended in collecting the material. Monographs and the works of specialists seldom pay, as we say. Translations and the editions of foreign works are rarely remunerative, although their publishers often pocket large sums from these enterprises. The contributors to our medical journals, even the ablest of them, are seldom adequately paid, a dollar a page, doled out in greenbacks, being the ordinary compensation. This is simply disreputable, and is, perhaps, one reason why so much of the periodical medical literature of the country is notoriously so indifferent. Self-respect should induce our better class of writers to demand higher rates of compensation, both for their own sake and for that of our literature. The rebuke lately administered by a distinguished English authoress to Edmund Yates, of London, is eminently applicable to the editors and publishers of our medical journals. Upon being offered ten guineas a week for a weekly portion of a novel for his magazine, she replied that her terms were double that amount, adding, "I have long since given up sacrificing my bread and butter in order to furnish gentlemen like yourself with cake and wine." Poor pay poor work is an old adage.

The difficulty of obtaining a publisher for one's work is often very great. If it had not been for James Webster, a poor bookseller of this city, it is questionable whether we should ever have had the benefit of the writings of Eberle; the first edition of Dunglison's Dictionary was issued at Boston, and I was myself compelled to travel all the way from Cincinnati to that city before I found a publisher for my work on pathological anatomy. The first volume of Drake's great work was issued, if I mistake not, only on condition that he should share with the publisher the responsibility of the undertaking.

18. CHARACTER OF AMERICAN MEDICAL LITERATURE.

From what precedes it is, I think, perfectly evident that America, in respect to her medical literature, as, indeed, in everything else, is able to take care of herself. What has hitherto retarded our progress was the reprint of foreign works which were thus brought into competition with our own, much to the detriment of their circulation and the reputation of their authors. If, to draw an illustration from my own department, Mr. Erichsen's Science and Art of Surgery had not been issued on this side of the Atlantic, my System of Surgery which, within the thirteen years since its publication, has passed through five large editions, would have been much more widely disseminated, and so also with the treatises of Ashhurst and Hamilton. The most popular surgical text book of our schools for upwards of a quarter of century was Druitt's Vade-Mecum, reprinted in this country under the title of the Principles and Practice of Surgery; a work written, not by a surgeon, but by an obstetric practitioner! Miller's books enjoyed for a number of years a very extensive circulation. Pirrie's Surgery never was a popular book with the American student and practitioner. That the circulation of Flint's Practice, despite its great popularity, has been much impaired by the reprint of Watson's Lectures, and of Aikin's Science and Art of Medicine, every one knows. On the other hand, it cannot be denied that the republication and dissemination of English works among us has exerted a most salutary influence upon the education of our physicians. If, fifty years ago, under the protection of an international copyright, we could have been thrown upon our own unaided efforts, there is no doubt that our native medical literature would long ago have attained the very highest pitch of excellence. Authors of great talent and attainment would have sprung up in every direction, feeling that they had every possible incentive to exert their best powers as observers, thinkers, and writers. One great obstacle still in our way is the use of foreign works as text-books in our schools, a practice as extensive as it is disgraceful to the profession and the country. If we cannot supply our institutions with elementary works on the different branches of medicine, the sooner we close their doors the better. How much jealousy, one of the most ignoble passions of the human mind, has to do with perpetuating this custom, so derogatory to our character as a great and otherwise independent profession, I will not stop to inquire.

If we compare the medical literature of America with that of Europe during the last hundred years, we shall have much cause for self-gratulation. In England, and, indeed, I may say on the continent, the exhibition prior to the close of the present century was, in truth, a most slender one, not at all flattering to the pride of our trans-Atlantic cousins. In Great Britain the works of Cullen and of Benjamin Bell were literally the first attempts at systematic medical authorship. Samuel Cooper did much to elevate the character of its surgical literature by the publication of his First Lines and of his great Dictionary of Surgery. Sir Astley Cooper produced immortal works, but they are not entitled to the name of systematic treatises. Druitt's Vade-Mecum was for a long time a text-book in the British schools. A quarter of a century has not elapsed since the appearance of the popular work of Mr. Erichsen. Holmes's Surgery is the joint production of many writers, not of one man. The works of Abernethy, of John and Charles Bell, of Colles, and of the Irish school generally, although replete in valuable matter, are not great national works. The latter part of the last century gave birth to the great works of Percivall Pott and of John Hunter, the founder of British Surgery. The able treatises of Stokes, Graves, and Watson on medicine, the Cyclopædia of Medicine by John Forbes and his colleagues, and the Library of Practical Medicine, edited by Alexander Tweedie, are comparatively recent productions, in advance, it is true, of anything of the kind in our own country.

In France, so boastful of its science and its arts, no work on surgery worthy of the name existed prior to the appearance of the treatise of Philip Boyer, in the early part of the present century. To this have been added, during the last twenty-five years, the works of Vidal and Nélaton. In practical medicine the most popular treatise is that of Valliex. The great French Dictionaries are well known. Germany has not, even now, any great work on surgery by a single author. The Handbuch der Chirurgie by Billroth and Pittha, in course of publication, is the joint labor of numerous writers. In medicine, physiology, pathology, pathological anatomy, and encyclography it enjoys an enviable reputation.

19. HOW AUTHORS DO THEIR WORK.

If any one asks, How, or by what means, these men accomplished their vast intellectual labors, the answer is an easy one. The busiest man, says the proverb, has the most leisure, and this assertion, paradoxical as it may appear, is perfectly true. The busy man is a systematic man; he utilizes the minutes, and lets the hours take care of themselves. No great literary work can be effected in any other way. But in some of the cases mentioned in this address, the result was greatly influenced by the leisure enjoyed by some of the writers. Thus, for example, Caldwell, as stated elsewhere, never had any practice, and had, therefore, perfect control of his time. Writing and lecturing were his ordinary occupations. The same may be said of Dunglison, and, in a considerable degree, of John Bell, Charles A. Lee, Martyn Paine, John W. Draper, Franklin Bache, and even of George B. Wood, who, although he was a hospital physician for upwards of a quarter of a century, never allowed private practice to interfere with his literary labors. It is different, very different, with a man actively engaged in practice, and dependent for his livelihood upon the number of daily visits he makes. Such a man, if he aspires to elaborate authorship, must work early and late, long, indeed, before ordinary mortals rise in the morning, and long after they have retired at night, or he will accomplish very little. To the question so often asked me, how I have been able to write so much, my answer invariably has been, because I have labored systematically while other men were asleep, smoking their cigar, lounging about the house, or spending the evenings in amusement. A vast amount of this work has been done in my carriage, in the daily rounds among my patients, not in actual writing, but in arranging and digesting my material, which, after reaching my office, I seized the earliest moment to commit to paper. In this manner a man may perform a large amount of literary labor in the twenty-four hours. The brain of a busy man is never idle. I have worked out many a sentence in my sleep.

Books, like their authors, have a period of adolescence, of mature growth, of decline, and even of actual dissolution.

Some fall stillborn from the press, many die in their infancy, a few attain to a vigorous manhood, and, now and then, one is fortunate enough to reach old age. The popularity of most works, however great at first, ceases long before the death of their authors. Many examples, illustrative of the truth of this remark, might be adduced, if time permitted, not only of works in our profession but in every other walk of life. Who of the present generation reads the works of Cooper, of Scott, or of Irving? Sad as this fate certainly is, it is, nevertheless, gratifying to know that a book, if good, although it may be short-lived, has been productive of benefit to the people for whose guidance and instruction it was written. Like its author, it served its day and generation, and can, therefore, afford to rest upon the shelf in honorable retirement, to share the fate of its predecessors and contemporaries. Now and then a student, more curious and inquisitive than the rest of his craft, anxious to look into the past, will be sure to exhume it, to shake the dust off its cover, and to pry into its contents, to see how the present compares with the past, to resuscitate forgotten ideas, and to revive the memory of the author. It is thus that men live in their works, and preserve the connecting links of medical literature and medical history.

20. MEDICAL BOOK PUBLISHERS.

I should not be doing justice to myself, nor, indeed, to my subject, if I were to omit to recall the names of some of the more prominent medical book publishers in this country, those men to whose discernment and enterprise we are indebted for the supply of our medical literature, native and foreign. If, occasionally, they do strike a good bargain with a native author, or fail to do justice to a British writer, in the way of compensation for the reprint of his works in the United States, it is only what happens every day in every other pursuit. As a body, they are just, honorable, high-toned. My own intercourse with them has always been highly agreeable; and the almost daily visit of a former colleague and excellent friend of mine, Professor Robley Dunglison, to the house of his publishers, during a period of a third of a century, showed the good opinion he entertained of their integrity, at the same time that it affords a beautiful proof of the warmth of their attachment to each other.

I have not been able to learn who ushered Wistar's Anatomy, the first systematic treatise in medicine ever issued on this continent by a native author, into the world; Dorsey's publisher was Edward Parker, and Kimbar & Howard, Market Street, Philadelphia. Thomas Dobson, in 1814, brought out a translation of Desault's surgical works, by Dr. E. Darrell Smith; and in 1819 James Webster performed the same office for Percivall Potts's celebrated chirurgical works. Alexander H. Stevens's translation of Baron Boyer's treatise on Surgical Diseases was published at New York. Early in the century a number of reprints of English works were issued by the Hartford press, as, for example, those of Charles Bell and John Abernethy on Surgery. The great publishing house, however, of the country was that originally of the Careys, descendants of Matthew Carey, an Irish gentleman of great intelligence and enterprise, who was himself engaged in the book business from 1783 till 1822. He then formed a partnership with his sons, which expired in 1825, when Carey, Lea & Carey came upon the stage, then Carey & Lea, Carey, Lea & Blanchard, Lea & Blanchard, and Blanchard & Lea, who, after a reign of fourteen years, were succeeded by Mr. Henry C. Lea, the eminent medical book publisher, who has ever since been his own master. From these respective firms a large majority of our native and reprinted medical works have emanated, and it affords me pleasure to add that they all have been fully rewarded for their labor and the investment of their capital.

The late Mr. John Grigg, a Welsh gentleman, who came to this country in his early youth, with only five shillings in his pocket, and retired from business a millionaire, was at one time extensively engaged in the publication of medical works. He brought out Eberle's Practice, Wood and Bache's United States Dispensatory, Wood's Practice, and other works since reproduced by Lippincott & Co. My acquaintance with Mr. Grigg began during my professional boyhood, when he stood sponsor for my translations of Bayle and Hollard's General Anatomy,

Hatin's Manual of Obstetrics, and Tavernier's Operative Surgery, followed soon after by my treatise on the Diseases and Injuries of the Bones and Joints. After my return to Philadelphia, in 1856, we again frequently met, and I always found him to be the same warm-hearted, impulsive gentleman he had been in early life, ever ready to extend his hand to a deserving man. He was, for a time, associated with Mr. Grambo in the publishing business, and, late in life, opened a private banking house. He often told me how much happier he had been with his five shillings than his millions.

Barrington & Haswell, once a prominent firm, issued a number of medical books; and Messrs. Lindsay & Blakiston have long enjoyed a wide reputation as publishers. The more eminent New York publishers of this class of works are the Woods, of Great Jones Street, and Appleton & Co., Broadway. The other cities of the Union have hardly done anything in this direction. Most of our authors, if they have any important or elaborate treatise on hand, anxious to secure for it a wide circulation, still turn their steps towards Philadelphia, as the religious devotee does towards Mecca.

I honor these men; for they deserve well of their country and of the outgoing century, for the services they have rendered to our medical literature. No doubt a meritorious author has occasionally left their doors in bitter disappointment, recalling the words of Gray as he cursed his fate:—

> "Full many a flower is born to blush unseen,
> And waste its sweetness on the desert air."

All men, fortunately or unfortunately, do not think alike.

Some of the members of the original house of the Careys and Leas are distinguished for their great talents and literary labors. Mathew Carey, the founder of the successive firms, was a copious writer, chiefly of pamphlets of a political and philanthropical character. Among these was a History of the Yellow Fever in 1793, of which four editions were published. Henry C. Carey has a world-wide reputation as a great writer on political economy, his works having been translated into nearly all the languages of Europe, and even into the Japanese. Isaac Lea, who was for many years a member of the firm, is universally known as a most copious contributor to the literature of natural science, almost every branch of which has been illustrated by his researches. As a conchologist he enjoys an unrivalled reputation on this continent. His son, Henry C. Lea, who now conducts the business, is widely known both in this country and in Europe, by his two learned works, Superstition and Force, and Studies in Church History.

21. MEDICAL LIBRARIES.

I propose, in conclusion, to say a few words respecting American Medical Libraries, Colleges, and Societies, as a kind of appendix to the history of our literature.

The oldest library in the United States is that of the Pennsylvania Hospital, founded in 1767, by Dr. Lloyd Zachary and Dr. Benjamin Morris. The present number of volumes, as I am informed by Dr. Frank Woodbury, is 12,000 in round numbers. The library of the College of Physicians of Philadelphia, instituted in 1787, contains nearly 19,000 volumes, independently of duplicates. Of this number nearly 5000 have been contributed by the munificent liberality of Dr. Samuel Lewis, of this city, who is actively engaged in the noble work of building up the library. The New York Hospital Library, as I am told by Dr. Purple, contains 10,000 volumes; the library of the New York Medical Journal Association, composed largely of medical periodicals, native and foreign, 3500 volumes; the Mott Memorial Library, 3000 volumes, many of them very rare and valuable. The Medical Department of Harvard University, as I am told by Dr. J. Collins Warren, contains about 7000 volumes. The Medical College of Ohio has less than 2000 volumes; the University of Louisville less than 5000; and the University of Virginia less than 4000. Dr. Otis writes me that the Army Medical Library at Washington City, established under the supervision of Surgeon-General Barnes, contains 42,000 bound volumes, and 40,000 pamphlets. By recent orders 4000 additional volumes are expected from Europe. These collections, respectable as they are, sink into insignificance in comparison with the 130,000 volumes in the Medical Library at Manchester, England.

The late Dr. John Redman Coxe had the finest library of the fathers of the profession in this country, if not in the world. He was engaged many years in collecting it, but had the bad taste to allow it to be sold under the hammer after his death. Dr. La Roche had the most complete collection of books on yellow and other fevers ever made in any country, which was also scattered to the winds a few years before he died. Such sacrifices are absolutely cruel, if not heart-rending. We may well ask, Where were the friends of the doctors, and the doctors themselves on these occasions?

My own library contains about 4500 volumes, rich in surgical literature. The library of Dr. Purple, of New York, consisting of 6000 volumes, contains a complete file of American journals, and the transactions of American Societies, with an extensive collection of English, Scotch, and Irish periodicals, and many choice editions of the Greek and Latin fathers. From a letter recently received from Dr. Purple, I learn that he has deposited all his periodical treasures, comprising upwards of 2000 volumes, in the library of the New York Academy of Medicine. My friend, Dr. Fisher, of Sing Sing, New York, has a valuable stock of ancient works. The library of Professor Stillé, comprising many choice volumes, especially in materia medica and therapeutics, was recently presented to the University of Pennsylvania.

Dr. Dunglison's library consisted of nearly 5000 volumes, and comprised the choicest works in almost every branch of medicine. It was particularly rich in works on physiology and the cognate sciences.

The late Dr. Hosack, of New York, the wealthiest member of the profession in his day in this country, had a library of 2500 volumes; Dr. John B. Beck, of 2000; Dr. Francis, of 3000; Dr. John Watson, of 2300. Dr. Watson's library was selected with much care and judgment, as well as at great cost. The historical part, a bequest from the eminent scholar and surgeon, is now in the New York Hospital, the remainder having been sold at auction. The library of the late Dr. Charles A. Luzenberg, of New Orleans, was one of the largest and choicest private collections of medical books ever made in this country. It was opulent in the writings of the fathers of the profession. What became of it after the death of the great physician and surgeon, in 1848, I am unable to state. The library of the late Dr. J. Collins Warren, of Boston, comprised 6000 volumes, rich in works on science and natural history.

22. MEDICAL SCHOOLS.

The first medical school on this continent was the University of Pennsylvania, founded in 1765, by Dr. John Morgan and Dr. William Shippen, with the powerful aid of Franklin, "Eripuit cælo fulmen sceptrumque tyrannus," the man who snatched the lightning from heaven, and the sceptre from tyrants. King's College, afterwards Columbia College, New York, was organized in 1768. The Medical Department of Harvard University went into operation in 1784; it was located at first at Cambridge, but in 1810 it was transferred to Boston, where it has remained ever since. The Medical School of Dartmouth College was founded, in 1798, by Nathan Smith, who was for twelve years sole professor, giving regular courses of lectures upon all the branches. The University of Maryland was established in 1807; the Medical Institution of New Haven in 1810; the Medical College of Ohio in 1818; Transylvania University at Lexington, Kentcuky, in 1819; the Medical College of the State of South Carolina at Charleston, in 1824; the Jefferson Medical College in 1825; the University of Louisville in 1837. Many of the earlier medical institutions had only a temporary existence. Some of them, as Rutgers Medical College of New York, and the Cincinnati Medical College, flashed, meteor-like, and then went under forever. Transylvania University, for a quarter of a century the great school of the West, with a world-wide fame of some of its teachers, and many prominent alumni, became extinct years ago. The causes of the downfall of most of these institutions have been dissensions in their faculties; now and then the charter happened to be defective; and in some instances the location was not well chosen. This was eminently true of the College of Physicians and Surgeons of the Western District of New York, established at Fairfield in 1812; of the Medical School at Pittsfield, Massachusetts; and of the Medical Department of Brown

University, Providence, Rhode Island, organized in 1821. No medical college can flourish for any length of time, even with the lowest grade of fees, unless it possesses superior facilities for clinical teaching and the study of practical anatomy. It was the want of such facilities that proved fatal to Transylvania University.

Of the number of medical schools at present in existence in the United States I am not accurately informed; it is probably not far short of eighty.

The number of chairs in the earlier history of our schools varied considerably. In the University of Pennsylvania the only teachers until 1768 were Morgan and Shippen, the latter having charge of anatomy, surgery, and midwifery until 1768, when Dr. Kuhn was added to the faculty, and the following year Dr. Rush, the former occupying the chair of medicine, and the latter that of chemistry. In the Medical School of Dartmouth College, Nathan Smith was for twelve years the sole professor, except during two sessions in which he was assisted by the department of chemistry. For the first quarter of the present century the best organized schools had, as a rule, only six chairs; subsequently most of them added another, the institutes of medicine. In the University of Pennsylvania there was no distinct chair of midwifery until 1810, the instruction in this department, prior to this period, having been given by the professor of anatomy. The fee for each professor was generally fifteen dollars in the older and more respectable schools, and the length of the session four months, with five or six lectures daily. Clinical instruction was generally delivered at the bedside, in the wards of the hospital, by the professors of medicine and surgery. Those schools that enjoyed no such advantages contented themselves with the occasional exhibition of stray cases of disease or injury. Gradually, as the necessity for this kind of instruction became more apparent, college clinics were established; an enterprise in which the Jefferson Medical College took the lead in this country, and to which much of her past and present prosperity is due. In the early progress of medical teaching in this country a number of the schools had a chair of botany, botany and mineralogy, or botany and natural history, as the Medical College at

Charleston, as late as 1824. The only wonder is that they did not also have instruction in astronomy and the occult sciences. During the last decade the number of chairs has been greatly multiplied, so that some of the schools have nearly as many instructors as pupils. Almost every conceivable organ of the body has its chair, except the umbilicus.

It was the custom, evidently borrowed from Europe, until within a comparatively recent period, in the schools of this country, for each professor to deliver an address at the opening of the session, introductory to his course of lectures, the first week of the session being usually consumed in this manner. Dr. Charles Caldwell, in his autobiography, in referring to his attendance upon the lectures in the University of Pennsylvania, states that the only introductory at that early day worth listening to was that of Rush, who had always a new one specially prepared for the occasion. One of the faculty, to quote the same authority, delivered annually, for years, the introductory lecture of his former preceptor, Dr. William Hunter, brother of the celebrated John Hunter, of London. It is said that the professor of chemistry, Dr. Woodhouse, pronounced the same introductory discourse for sixteen consecutive years, and when asked why he did not occasionally write a new one, he answered, "Because I always discover new beauty and excellence in the old one." I recollect listening, many years ago, to an introductory lecture in a western school, copied almost verbatim from Quain's Anatomy, then little known in this country. Such bare-faced acts would, of course, not be tolerated at the present day. Instead of each professor delivering an introductory address at the opening of the college session, this duty is now very wisely intrusted to one member of the faculty, and the consequence is that the student gains nearly one week of useful instruction.

23. MEDICAL SOCIETIES.

When it is remembered that the great objects of medical societies are to promote harmony and good feeling among their members, to regulate the practice of medicine, and to prevent quackery, one of the great evils of a country, it is not surprising that the attention of our medical forefathers should have been directed at an early period to the establishment of such institutions. Leaving out of the question several abortive efforts of this kind in this city, immediately prior to the revolution, we find that the first successful one was the Medical Society of New Jersey, which was organized in 1766, and which held its one hundred and ninth meeting at Atlantic City last May. This Society, strange to say, possesses the power, by an act of the State legislature, of conferring the degree of doctor of medicine, instead of a license certificate, upon physicians desirous of practising in that commonwealth without the proper qualifications from an authorized medical college. The Massachusetts Medical Society was incorporated by an act of the legislature in 1781, and organized the following June by the election to its presidency of Dr. Edward A. Holyoke, of Salem, famous alike as an accomplished physician and a noble citizen, who died in 1829 at the age of one hundred years. The College of Physicians of Philadelphia was founded in 1789, and consists of fellows and associates, nearly two hundred in number, and embracing nearly all the prominent physicians of the city. The College possesses a rich library and an excellent museum of healthy and morbid anatomy, the former embracing the valuable collection of Professor Hyrtl of Vienna, and the latter the collection of the late Professor Mütter, who by will donated it to the College along with $30,000 for the increase and preservation of the museum. The Connecticut Medical Society was organized in 1793; the Medical Society of the State of New York in 1806; and the American Medical Association in 1846, its founder having been Professor N. S. Davis, then of Binghamton, New York, and now of Chicago, and its first President, Dr. Nathaniel Chapman, the celebrated Professor of Medicine in the University of Pennsylvania. The first annual meeting was held at Baltimore in May, 1848. Dr. William B. Atkinson, of this city, has for many years been its Secretary. Every State and almost every Territory in the Union now has its medical Society; and it would be difficult to over-estimate the amount of good which these institutions are doing in elevating the character, dignity, and usefulness of the American medical profession. Our medical literature, as stated elsewhere, receives annually important contributions from these sources.

A medical society, embracing under-graduates during their attendance upon lectures, was organized in this city, in 1821, and for a number of years successfully conducted, its first president having been Professor Dewees, and its first orator Professor Chapman. It consisted of senior, honorary, and junior members, and reading and discussing papers on medical topics formed its chief exercises. A society, conducted upon a similar plan, existed for some years in the University of Louisville, and was productive of much good, as it afforded students an opportunity of displaying their knowledge of medicine, and their ability as debaters. I throw out the hint whether it would not be well to form such an association in connection with this school.

24. CUSTOMS AND PRACTICES.

At the commencement of the revolutionary war the population of the American colonies was about 3,000,000, which, towards the close of the century, had increased to 4,500,000. The number of physicians in active practice at the outbreak of the rebellion was, as nearly as can be estimated at a rough guess, about 3000. Of these, the great majority had never received a medical degree, while the remainder, with few exceptions, had obtained their education abroad, chiefly at the University of Edinburgh, at that time and for a long while subsequently the most renowned school in the world. Morgan, Shippen, Kuhn, Rush, McDowell, Hosack, Miller, Mitchill, Gibson, and many others of note, completed their studies in that great seminary of medicine. Charleston, South Carolina, had at one time upwards of a dozen graduates hailing from the Scottish capital. It was then as much the custom for American students to go to Edinburgh in quest of knowledge as it now is for them to go to Paris, Berlin, or Vienna. The period of study was longer in those days than it is at present, and the pupil was required to have a greater amount of preliminary education. Without some knowledge of the Greek and Latin languages no youth was permitted to pass the portals of a medical college. Kuhn studied six or seven and Rush nine years before they entered upon the active duties of their profession. The theses were written in Latin, and defended publicly on commencement day.

In the early practice of the country, physicians compounded their own prescriptions, as is, indeed, still the custom with practitioners in the rural districts and smaller towns. Dr. John Morgan, the founder of the University of Pennsylvania, was the first to attempt to reform this custom, which, as a consequence, was gradually abolished in Philadelphia and other prominent cities. Educated pharmacists, who now very properly have charge of this business, abound in this country, thus relieving medical men of a vast amount of drudgery and responsibility. No medical journals existed, and the medical libraries were of the most slender character.

The fashion, which prevailed for so many centuries, of wearing a wig and carrying a gold-headed cane, was adopted by some of our earlier physicians. The last one of any distinction who adhered to the custom, always, one would suppose, more honored in the breach than in the observance, was Dr. Kuhn, Professor of Medicine in the University of Pennsylvania, who, in addition, carried a gold snuff-box, and wore gold knee and shoe buckles. The last physician of any note in Great Britain who made use of the gold-headed cane was the celebrated Dr. Matthew Baillie, a nephew of the Hunters, and the author of the work on morbid anatomy alluded to in a previous part of this discourse. After his death, his widow presented this precious relic to the Royal College of Physicians of London, in whose possession it still remains. Physick was the last of his race in this city to wear a queue and to powder his hair; a practice at one time almost universal in this country among well-bred gentlemen. The medical doctrines prevalent in the United States a century ago were, for a long time, those taught by Dr. Cullen in his lectures in the University of Edinburgh and in his Physiology, his First Lines of the Practice of Medicine, and in his Materia Medica. When Rush, a pupil of the Edinburgh school, entered upon his brilliant career, he became a strong advocate of blood-letting and other heroic remedies, a practice which obtained among our physicians until a third of a century ago. The doctrine of solidism had at one time an exclusive reign both in Europe and in this country, where its last advocates were Nathaniel Chapman, Charles Caldwell, and John P. Harrison, men who adhered with bull-dog tenacity to their foolish creed. When I entered upon the study of the profession Broussaism, which taught that most diseases were located in the mucous membrane of the alimentary canal, and could be most readily and effectually cured with ptisans, gumwater, and leeches, was just coming into vogue, its great advocate on this side of the Atlantic being the late Dr. Samuel Jackson, Professor of the Institutes of Medicine in the University of Pennsylvania. John Esten Cooke, of Lexington, Kentucky, asserted that all maladies depended upon obstruction of the portal circulation, or disorder of the liver, and contended with all the ardor of a devotee that the only remedies necessary for their relief were rhubarb, aloes, and calomel, or the R. A. C. pill, as it was called by him and his followers. Benjamin W. Dudley, the famous lithotomist, one of the founders of Transylvania University, and a colleague of Cooke, had unbounded faith in the treatment of diseases, surgical as well as medical, by the use of bran gruel, blue milk, and boiled turnips, calomel, tartar emetic, and absolute and protracted rest. These heroic measures, the offspring of great men's brains gone mad, gradually gave way to the practice of almost unconditional stimulation, which for upwards of a quarter of a century has enslaved the professional mind of Europe and this country, and which, without exaggeration, it is safe to say, counts its victims annually by thousands. Every age has its characteristics. If I were permitted to express an opinion of those of the present day, I should say that they consisted in a reckless spirit of experimentation, in loose observation, in unfounded statements, in inefficient practice, and in hasty generalization. Our times abound emphatically in false facts.

25. SPECIALISTS.

When I entered the profession there were no specialists, as they are now called, a class of men devoted mainly to the practice of some particular branch of the healing art. Indeed, it is only within the last twenty-five years that this class of medical men have acquired any decided prominence. From small beginnings they have grown into a formidable body, exercising a wide-spread influence, and threatening the general practitioner with destruction by robbing him of his business and emoluments. In our large cities and towns their number is legion. The physician who in this country led the way in this innovation was the late Dr. Horace Green, of New York, who, for many years, enjoyed an unrivalled reputation as a "throat doctor;" and such was his success that numerous followers have since sprung up in all parts of the world. I do not feel inclined to break a lance with the specialists; but I submit, with all deference, whether the general practitioner, if thoroughly educated and fully up to the times, is not better qualified to do justice to his patients than the man who limits himself in his practice to the affections of one or two organs whether, in other words, the mind does not enlarge and expand in the one case, so as to be able to take a more comprehensive view of a disease, while in the other it has a tendency to dwarf it or to tie it down within a very narrow compass. In this country nearly every medical man, either at the outset of his professional life or after he has been for some time engaged in its active exercise, almost instinctively drops into some specialty, as a mere matter of choice, in the pursuit of which, without an abandonment of his other business, he gradually acquires skill and fame, and yet never aspires to be considered as a specialist; nay, in fact, would regard it as an insult to be called one. Dentists can hardly be said to be specialists; it is true, the more refined and conscientious confine themselves strictly to the treatment of the teeth; but so much of their work is mechanical that no general practitioner of medicine, at all extensively occupied, could give it the requisite attention. Every body, sooner or later, has need of this class of professional men, for every adult has thirty-two teeth, which, however sound, require occasional supervision to keep them in order. On the other hand, comparatively few persons suffer from cataract or cancer of the eye, morbid growths of the larynx, diseases of the ear, or ulceration of the uterus. I venture to affirm that Dudley, who was a general practitioner of medicine and surgery, extracted a stone from the bladder with as much dexterity as any specialist that ever lived; and I am quite sure that no oculist, so called, one exclusively devoted to the practice of ophthalmic medicine and surgery, ever extracted a cataract with more skill than the Emeritus-professor of Anatomy in this school. I am sure it requires only the smallest amount of brains to make a specialist. I cannot forbear here to quote the felicitous commentary of Dr. Barnes, of London, upon this subject, as it admirably illustrates the tendency of the age: "I have recently," he says, "been honored by a visit from a lady of typical modern intelligence, who consulted me about a fibroid tumor of the uterus; and, lest I should stray beyond my business, she was careful to tell me that Dr. Brown-Séquard had charge of her nervous system, that Dr. Williams attended to her lungs, that her abdominal organs were intrusted to Sir William Gull, that Spencer Wells looked after her rectum, and that Dr. Walshe had her heart. If some adventurous doctor should determine to have a new specialty, and open an institution for the treatment of diseases of the umbilicus, the only region which is unappropriated, I think I could promise more than one patient." Dr. Barnes is in error. The vermiform appendix has no specialist.

26. CLOSING REMARKS.

No one who has been an attentive observer of the progress in our profession during the last third of a century can have failed to be struck with wonder and amazement at the vast changes and improvements that have been made in all its branches. Chemistry and physiology have been so completely revolutionized as to render it difficult to believe that they are the same sciences; the books on these subjects, written at or prior to that period, once proudly pointed at as the text-books in our schools, are as obsolete as if they had never had any existence. In the practical branches—medicine, surgery, and midwifery—many new channels have been opened and vast improvements effected, all tending to the amelioration of suffering, the prolongation of life, and the dignity and usefulness of the healing art. The march is still onward and upward, more rapidly and more earnestly than ever before, but whether we shall ever discover the Elixir of Life, at one time, like the Philosopher's Stone, an object of so much research and anxious inquiry, it is not for us mortals to know. Honest and earnest seekers after truth, let us work and hope, and thus fulfil our destiny, as the Great Author of the universe has appointed it.

I have thus, my young friends, shown, if I do not greatly err, that we have a medical literature, based upon a broad and solid foundation; a literature full of vigor and inspiration, honorable alike to the profession and to the nation. I have portrayed to you, perhaps too feebly, one of the noble legacies bequeathed to us by our forefathers. Let us, their heirs, cherish their memories, and strive to render ourselves worthy of our inheritance. Many of the laborers enumerated in this address have gone to their rest, but their works remain and they live in the affection and esteem of their successors. When another century shall have rolled by, let it be said of you, as we now say of those who have preceded us, that you have been worthy of your age and country, and of your renowned ancestry. Let your children and children's children weave for you a chaplet of evergreens as you now weave one for the brows of the medical sages and heroes of the expiring year. May the voice never be heard in the land which the Lord God has given us as our dwelling place: "Ichabod! Ichabod, thy glory has departed!"